THE INTUITIVE EATING COOKBOOK

Transform Your Relationship with Food, Ten Principles for Nourishing a Healthy Connection with The Intuitive Eating Cookbook with 50 Mouthwatering Recipes

Jessica M. Steven

Table of contents

INTRODUCTION

Introducing "The Intuitive Eating Cookbook: Nourish Your Body, Mind, and Spirit" a culinary journey that goes beyond the plate to transform your relationship with food. In this cookbook, we embrace the principles of intuitive eating, guiding you to listen to your body's wisdom, honor your hunger, and find satisfaction in every meal.

Drawing from the core principles of intuitive eating, this cookbook offers a refreshing approach to nourishing your body. It's not about strict diets or rigid meal plans; instead, it's about embracing a mindset of self-care, compassion, and mindfulness when it comes to food.

"The Intuitive Eating Cookbook" is more than just a collection of recipes; it's a guide to cultivating a healthier and more joyful relationship with food. Each recipe is designed to help you tune into your body's hunger and fullness cues, and discover the satisfaction that comes from eating mindfully and intuitively.

With over 100 delicious and nutritious recipes, this cookbook offers something for everyone, whether you're a seasoned chef or just starting out in the kitchen. From vibrant salads to hearty soups, satisfying mains to indulgent desserts, each recipe is designed to nourish your body, mind, and spirit.

Join us on this journey to rediscover the joy of eating and transform your relationship with food. Let "The Intuitive Eating Cookbook" be your guide to a healthier, happier, and more fulfilling way of nourishing yourself.

CHAPTER ONE

Embracing Intuitive Eating: Rejecting the Diet Mentality for a Healthier Relationship with Food

In a world inundated with fad diets and weight-loss trends, the concept of intuitive eating stands out as a refreshing and sustainable approach to nourishing our bodies. At its core, intuitive eating encourages us to reject the diet mentality and instead tune into our body's natural hunger and fullness cues. It's about honoring our cravings, respecting our bodies, and ultimately finding joy and satisfaction in eating.

The diet mentality, on the other hand, is deeply ingrained in our society. We're bombarded with messages that tell us we need to restrict, count calories,
and adhere to strict meal plans in order to achieve the "perfect" body. This mindset not only fosters feelings of guilt and shame around food but also ignores the individuality of our bodies and their needs.

Intuitive eating offers a different perspective. It's about trusting our bodies to guide us towards the foods that will truly nourish us, both physically and emotionally. This means letting go of the idea that certain foods are "good" or "bad" and instead focusing on how different foods make us feel.

One of the key principles of intuitive eating is rejecting the notion of "forbidden" foods. When we label foods as off-limits, we only increase their appeal and set ourselves up for feelings of failure and guilt when we inevitably indulge. Intuitive eating encourages us to enjoy all foods in moderation, without judgment.

Another important aspect of intuitive eating is learning to distinguish between physical hunger and other types of hunger, such as emotional or boredom eating. By paying attention to our body's cues, we can better understand what our true needs are and respond to them accordingly.

But perhaps the most powerful aspect of intuitive eating is its focus on self-compassion. It's about treating ourselves with kindness and understanding, even when we don't always make the healthiest choices. It's about recognizing that our worth is not determined by the number on the scale or the size of our jeans.

intuitive eating offers us a path to freedom from the diet mentality that so often plagues our relationship with food. It's about trusting our bodies,
honoring our cravings, and finding joy in eating. By rejecting the diet mentality and embracing intuitive eating, we can cultivate a healthier, more sustainable relationship with food and ourselves.

CHAPTER TWO
Honoring Your Hunger: The Key to a Healthy Relationship with Food

In a world obsessed with diets and weight loss, the simple act of honoring your hunger can seem revolutionary. Yet, listening to your body's signals and responding with nourishing food is a fundamental aspect of intuitive eating, a philosophy that encourages a healthy relationship with food and your body.

Honoring your hunger means acknowledging when you're physically hungry and responding to that hunger in a way that respects your body's needs. It's about recognizing that hunger is a natural, biological signal that should not be ignored or suppressed.

One of the core principles of intuitive eating is rejecting the diet mentality, which often teaches us to fear hunger and view it as something to be avoided. Instead, intuitive eating encourages us to trust our bodies and believe that they know what they need to thrive.

When we honor our hunger, we are better able to tune into our body's cues and eat in a way that feels satisfying and nourishing. This means eating when we're hungry, rather than waiting until we're ravenous, and stopping when we're full, rather than feeling obligated to clean our plates.

Honoring your hunger also means being mindful of the types of foods you choose to eat. It's about choosing foods that will truly nourish you and give you the energy you need to live your life to the fullest. This might mean opting for whole, unprocessed foods that are rich in nutrients,

rather than processed foods that are high in empty calories.

But honoring your hunger is about more than just what you eat; it's also about how you eat. It's about taking the time to sit down and savor your meals, rather than rushing through them. It's about paying attention to how different foods make you feel, both physically and emotionally, and adjusting your eating habits accordingly.

In conclusion, honoring your hunger is a powerful act of self-care that can help you develop a healthy relationship with food and your body. By listening to your body's signals and responding with compassion and respect, you can nourish yourself in a way that feels satisfying and sustainable.

CHAPTER THREE
Making Peace with Food: Embracing Freedom and Joy in Eating

In a culture that often demonizes certain foods and glorifies others, making peace with food can seem like a radical act of rebellion. But for those practicing intuitive eating, it's a fundamental principle that can lead to a healthier, more balanced relationship with food and your body.

Making peace with food means letting go of the idea that certain foods are "good" or "bad" and instead embracing all foods as nourishing and satisfying in their own way. It's about rejecting the restrictive rules and guilt that often accompany eating and instead focusing on pleasure, satisfaction, and nourishment.

One of the key tenets of intuitive eating is rejecting the diet mentality, which teaches us to view certain foods as off-limits and to feel guilty when we indulge in them. Instead, intuitive eating encourages us to trust our bodies to guide us towards the foods that will truly nourish us, both physically and emotionally.

When we make peace with food, we give ourselves permission to enjoy all foods in moderation, without judgment or guilt. This doesn't mean eating whatever we want, whenever we want; it means listening to our bodies' hunger and fullness cues and responding with compassion and respect.

Making peace with food also means recognizing that food is more than just fuel; it's a source of pleasure, comfort, and connection. It's about savoring the flavors and textures of our favorite foods, and enjoying the experience of eating without guilt or shame.

But perhaps most importantly, making peace with food is about recognizing that our worth is not determined by what or how much we eat. It's about separating our value as individuals from the foods we choose to eat, and learning to treat ourselves with kindness and compassion, regardless of our food choices.

In conclusion, making peace with food is a powerful act of self-love and self-care that can lead to a healthier, more balanced relationship with food and your body. By rejecting the diet mentality and embracing all foods as nourishing and satisfying, you can find freedom and joy in eating, and cultivate a sense of peace and contentment in your relationship with food.

CHAPTER FOUR
Challenging the Food Police: Liberating Yourself from Food Judgment

In a world filled with food rules and regulations, challenging the food police can be a liberating act of self-compassion and empowerment. The food police are the voices in our heads – and often in our society – that dictate what we should and shouldn't eat, based on arbitrary rules and standards. These voices can lead to guilt, shame, and anxiety around food, ultimately harming our relationship with eating and our bodies.

Challenging the food police means rejecting these harmful messages and instead embracing a more mindful and intuitive approach to eating.

It's about trusting your body to guide you towards the foods that will truly nourish you, both physically and emotionally, and letting go of the judgment and guilt that often accompany food choices.

One of the key principles of intuitive eating is rejecting the diet mentality, which is perpetuated by the food police. This mentality teaches us to view certain foods as "good" and others as "bad," and to feel guilty when we indulge in the "bad" foods. Instead, intuitive eating encourages us to enjoy all foods in moderation, without judgment or guilt.

Challenging the food police also means challenging the idea that our worth is tied to our food choices. It's about recognizing that our value as individuals is not determined by what or how much we eat, and learning to treat ourselves with kindness and compassion, regardless of our food choices.

But perhaps most importantly, challenging the food police is about reclaiming your power and autonomy when it comes to eating. It's about listening to your body's hunger and fullness cues, and responding with self-compassion and respect. It's about recognizing that you are the expert on your own body, and trusting yourself to make choices that are truly nourishing and satisfying.

In conclusion, challenging the food police is a radical act of self-love and empowerment that can lead to a healthier, more balanced relationship with food and your body. By rejecting harmful food rules and embracing a more intuitive approach to eating, you can free yourself from guilt, shame, and anxiety around food, and find joy and freedom in eating once again.

CHAPTER FIVE
Feel Your Fullness: The Art of Eating Mindfully and Satisfying Your Hunger

In a world filled with distractions and hectic schedules, it's easy to overlook one of the most important aspects of eating: feeling your fullness. The concept of feeling your fullness is central to intuitive eating, a philosophy that encourages us to listen to our bodies' hunger and fullness cues in order to nourish ourselves in a way that is satisfying and sustainable.

Feeling your fullness means being aware of your body's signals and stopping eating when you are satisfied, rather than when your plate is empty or when you feel uncomfortably full.

It's about honoring your body's natural wisdom and trusting that it knows when it has had enough.

One of the key principles of intuitive eating is rejecting the diet mentality, which often teaches us to ignore our body's signals and instead follow external rules and guidelines about when and how much to eat. Instead, intuitive eating encourages us to trust our bodies to guide us towards the foods and quantities that will truly nourish us.

Practicing feeling your fullness can take time and practice, especially if you're used to eating quickly or eating past the point of fullness. One helpful strategy is to eat slowly and mindfully, paying attention to the flavors, textures, and sensations of each bite. This can help you tune into your body's signals and recognize when you are starting to feel satisfied.

Another helpful strategy is to check in with yourself periodically throughout the meal and ask yourself how hungry or full you are on a scale of 1 to 10. This can help you become more aware of your body's signals and make more informed choices about when to continue eating and when to stop.

But perhaps the most important aspect of feeling your fullness is learning to trust yourself and your body's wisdom. It's about recognizing that you are the expert on your own body, and that only you can determine when and how much to eat. By practicing feeling your fullness, you can develop a healthier, more balanced relationship with food and your body, and find joy and satisfaction in eating once again.

CHAPTER SIX
Discover the Satisfaction Factor: How to Find Joy and Fulfillment in Eating

In our fast-paced world, it's easy to overlook the importance of satisfaction in eating. Yet, the satisfaction factor is a crucial component of intuitive eating, a philosophy that encourages us to honor our hunger, respect our fullness, and find joy and fulfillment in the eating experience.

Discovering the satisfaction factor means finding pleasure and enjoyment in the foods we eat, as well as in the act of eating itself. It's about recognizing that food is not just fuel, but also a source of pleasure, comfort, and connection.

One of the key principles of intuitive eating is rejecting the diet mentality, which often teaches us to view food as the enemy and to deprive ourselves of the foods we love in the name of health or weight loss. Instead, intuitive eating encourages us to enjoy all foods in moderation and to savor the flavors and textures of our meals. Practicing the satisfaction factor can take many forms. It might mean exploring new foods and flavors, or rediscovering old favorites. It might mean taking the time to prepare and savor a home-cooked meal, or enjoying a meal with loved ones and engaging in meaningful conversation.

One important aspect of the satisfaction factor is learning to eat mindfully. This means paying attention to the flavors, textures, and sensations of each bite, and eating slowly and attentively. Mindful eating can help us tune into our body's signals of hunger and fullness, and can enhance our enjoyment of the eating experience.

But perhaps the most important aspect of the satisfaction factor is learning to trust our bodies and our own internal cues. It's about recognizing that we are the experts on our own bodies, and that only we can determine what foods and eating habits truly satisfy us.

In conclusion, discovering the satisfaction factor is a powerful tool for developing a healthier, more balanced relationship with food and our bodies. By honoring our hunger, respecting our fullness, and finding joy and fulfillment in eating, we can cultivate a positive and sustainable approach to nutrition and find greater satisfaction in all areas of our lives.

CHAPTER SEVEN
Coping with Your Feelings: Finding Healthy Alternatives to Emotional Eating

Food has long been associated with comfort and emotional support. However, relying on food to cope with our feelings can lead to a host of issues, including unhealthy eating habits and a strained relationship with food. Learning to cope with your feelings without using food is an important skill that can help you develop a healthier relationship with eating and improve your overall well-being.

One of the key principles of intuitive eating is learning to recognize and honor your feelings without using food as a coping mechanism. This means being mindful of your emotions and finding alternative ways to address them that don't involve eating.

One effective way to cope with your feelings without using food is to practice mindfulness. Mindfulness involves being present in the moment and observing your thoughts and feelings without judgment. By practicing mindfulness, you can learn to acknowledge your emotions without feeling the need to suppress them with food.

Another helpful strategy is to engage in activities that help you relax and unwind, such as yoga, meditation, or deep breathing exercises. These activities can help you manage stress and anxiety without turning to food for comfort.

It can also be helpful to find healthy outlets for your emotions, such as talking to a friend or therapist, journaling, or engaging in creative activities like painting or dancing. These activities can help you express and process your feelings in a constructive way.

But perhaps the most important aspect of coping with your feelings without using food is learning to be kind and compassionate towards yourself. It's okay to have emotions, and it's okay to feel them. By treating yourself with compassion and finding healthy ways to cope with your feelings, you can develop a healthier relationship with food and improve your overall emotional well-being.

In conclusion, learning to cope with your feelings without using food is an important skill that can help you develop a healthier relationship with eating and improve your overall well-being. By practicing mindfulness, engaging in relaxing activities, finding healthy outlets for your emotions, and being kind to yourself, you can learn to address your feelings in a constructive way that doesn't involve turning to food for comfort.

CHAPTER EIGHT
Respect Your Body: Embracing Self-Acceptance and Body Positivity

Respecting your body is a fundamental aspect of intuitive eating, a philosophy that encourages us to honor our bodies' needs and cues in order to develop a healthy and sustainable relationship with food. It's about recognizing that our bodies are unique and deserving of care and respect, regardless of their shape or size. One of the key principles of intuitive eating is rejecting the diet mentality, which often teaches us to view our bodies as enemies to be conquered and controlled. Instead, intuitive eating encourages us to trust our bodies and listen to their signals of hunger, fullness, and satisfaction.

Respecting your body means accepting and appreciating it for all that it is, rather than focusing on perceived flaws or imperfections. It's about recognizing that our bodies are capable of amazing things and that they deserve to be treated with kindness and compassion.

One important aspect of respecting your body is learning to practice self-care. This means nourishing your body with healthy foods, getting regular exercise, and getting enough rest and relaxation. It also means listening to your body's signals and responding with compassion and respect.

Another important aspect of respecting your body is learning to practice body positivity. Body positivity is about accepting and loving your body as it is, regardless of societal standards or ideals. It's about recognizing that beauty comes in all shapes and sizes, and that our worth is not determined by our appearance.

But perhaps the most important aspect of respecting your body is learning to be kind to yourself. It's about recognizing that you are worthy of love and respect, regardless of your size or shape. By practicing self-compassion and treating yourself with kindness, you can develop a healthier and more positive relationship with your body.

In conclusion, respecting your body is an essential component of intuitive eating and can lead to a more positive and fulfilling relationship with food and your body. By rejecting the diet mentality, practicing self-care, embracing body positivity, and being kind to yourself, you can learn to respect and appreciate your body for all that it is.

CHAPTER NINE
Exercise: Feel the Difference in Your Mind, Body, and Spirit

Exercise is often seen as a means to an end, a way to burn calories or change the shape of our bodies. However, when approached from a place of self-care and self-compassion, exercise can be a powerful tool for improving not just our physical health, but also our mental and emotional well-being.

One of the key principles of intuitive eating is making peace with movement. This means letting go of the idea that exercise is a punishment for eating or a way to manipulate our bodies, and instead embracing it as a way to honor and care for ourselves.

When we exercise in a way that feels good and nourishing to our bodies, we can experience a host of benefits beyond just physical fitness. Exercise has been shown to improve mood, reduce anxiety and depression, and increase overall feelings of well-being. It can also improve sleep, boost energy levels, and enhance cognitive function.

One of the reasons exercise is so beneficial for our mental health is because it releases endorphins, chemicals in the brain that act as natural painkillers and mood elevators. This is often referred to as the "runner's high," but any form of exercise that gets your heart rate up can have similar effects.

But perhaps the most powerful aspect of exercise is the way it can help us connect with our bodies. When we exercise mindfully, paying attention to how our bodies feel and responding with compassion and respect, we can develop a deeper appreciation for our bodies and all they are capable of.

In conclusion, exercise is a powerful tool for improving not just our physical health, but also our mental and emotional well-being. By approaching exercise from a place of self-care and self-compassion, and focusing on how it makes us feel rather than how it makes us look, we can experience the true transformative power of movement.

CHAPTER TEN
Honor Your Health: Embracing Gentle Nutrition for a Balanced and Nourishing Diet

In the world of nutrition, it's easy to get caught up in strict rules and rigid guidelines about what we should and shouldn't eat. However, when it comes to honoring our health, a more gentle and flexible approach to nutrition can be both more sustainable and more nourishing.

Gentle nutrition is a key principle of intuitive eating, a philosophy that encourages us to listen to our bodies' hunger and fullness cues and eat in a way that is satisfying and sustainable. It's about finding a balance between nourishing our bodies with healthy foods and allowing ourselves to enjoy the foods we love without guilt or restriction.

One of the key aspects of gentle nutrition is focusing on the overall quality of our diet, rather than getting bogged down in specific nutrients or calorie counts. This means emphasizing whole, minimally processed foods, such as fruits, vegetables, whole grains, and lean proteins, while still allowing ourselves to enjoy treats and indulgences in moderation.

Another important aspect of gentle nutrition is learning to tune into our bodies' signals and eat in a way that feels good and satisfying. This might mean eating when we're hungry and stopping when we're full, rather than following strict meal times or portion sizes.

Gentle nutrition also encourages us to be mindful of how different foods make us feel, both physically and emotionally. For example, we might notice that certain foods give us energy and make us feel good, while others might leave us feeling sluggish or bloated. By paying attention to these cues, we can make more informed choices about what to eat.

But perhaps the most important aspect of gentle nutrition is learning to approach food with a sense of curiosity and openness. It's about recognizing that there is no one-size-fits-all approach to nutrition, and that what works for one person may not work for another. By being open to trying new foods and eating in a way that feels good and satisfying, we can develop a healthier and more balanced relationship with food and our bodies.

In conclusion, honoring your health with gentle nutrition is about finding a balance between nourishing your body with healthy foods and allowing yourself to enjoy the foods you love without guilt or restriction. By approaching nutrition with a sense of flexibility and openness, you can develop a more sustainable and nourishing approach to eating that honors your health and well-being.

BREAKFAST RECIPES TO KICKSTART YOUR DAY

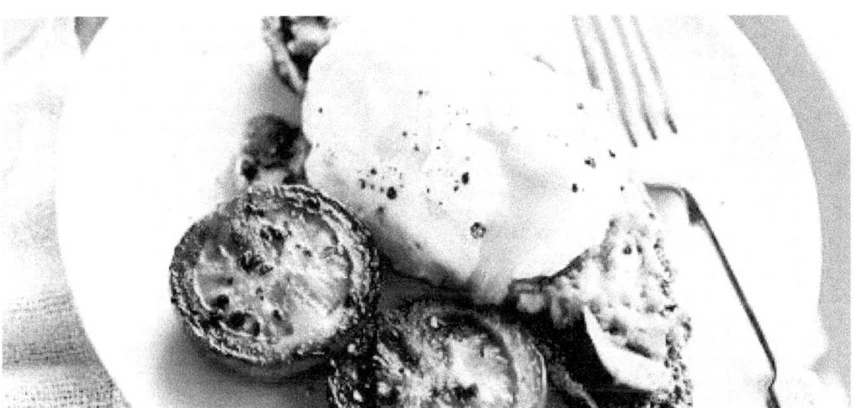

Avocado Toast with Poached Egg

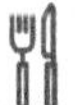 1 servings   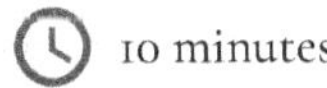 10 minutes

INGREDIENTS

1 ripe avocado

1 egg

1 slice whole grain
bread

Salt and pepper to taste

NUTRITIONAL VALUE

300 calories,

15g protein,

20g fat,

25g carbohydrates,

10g fiber

DIRECTIONS

1. 1. Toast the bread until golden brown.
2. 2. Mash the avocado in a bowl and season with salt and pepper.
3. 3. Poach the egg in simmering water until cooked to your liking.
4. 4. Spread the mashed avocado on the toast and top with the poached egg.
5. 5. Season with additional salt and pepper if desired.

NOTES

This recipe combines creamy avocado with a perfectly poached egg on top of crunchy whole grain toast, creating a satisfying and nutritious breakfast.

16

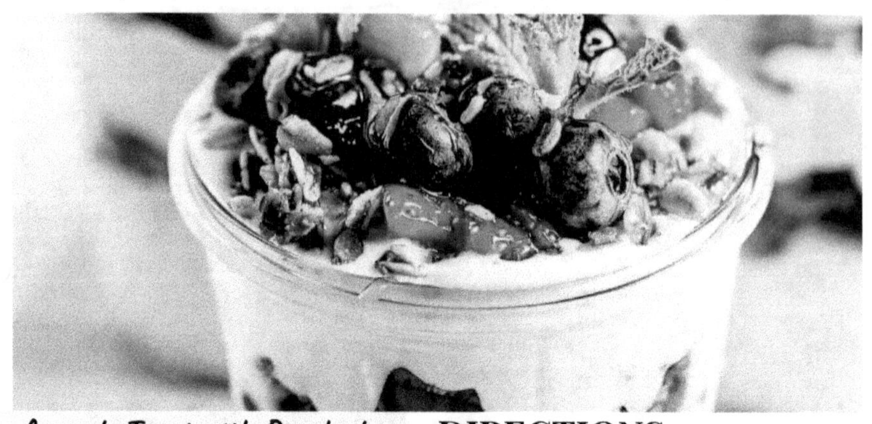

Avocado Toast with Poached Egg

 1 servings   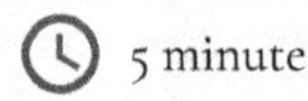 5 minutes

INGREDIENTS

1/2 cup Greek yogurt

1/4 cup granola

1/4 cup mixed berries

(strawberries,

blueberries,

raspberries)

NUTRITIONAL VALUE

250 calories,

15g protein,

8g fat,

30g carbohydrates,

5g fiber

DIRECTIONS

1. 1. In a glass, layer the Greek yogurt, granola, and berries.
2. 2. Repeat the layers until all ingredients are used.
3. 3. Serve immediately and enjoy!

NOTES

Layers of creamy Greek yogurt, crunchy granola, and sweet berries make this parfait a delicious and nutritious way to start your day.

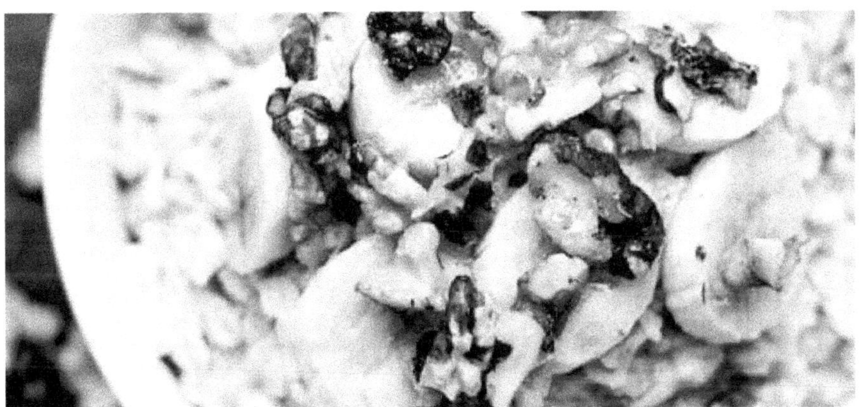

Oatmeal with Almond Butter and Banana

 1 servings  10 minutes

INGREDIENTS

1/2 cup rolled oats

1 cup water or milk

1 tablespoon almond butter

1/2 banana, sliced

DIRECTIONS

1. 1. In a saucepan, bring the water or milk to a boil.
2. 2. Stir in the oats and reduce heat to low.
3. 3. Cook for 5 minutes, stirring occasionally, until the oats are creamy.
4. 4. Stir in the almond butter until well combined.
5. 5. Transfer the oatmeal to a bowl and top with banana slices.

NUTRITIONAL VALUE

350 calories,

10g protein,

12g fat,

50g carbohydrates,

8g fiber

NOTES

This oatmeal is made with creamy almond butter and topped with fresh banana slices for a hearty and satisfying breakfast.

18

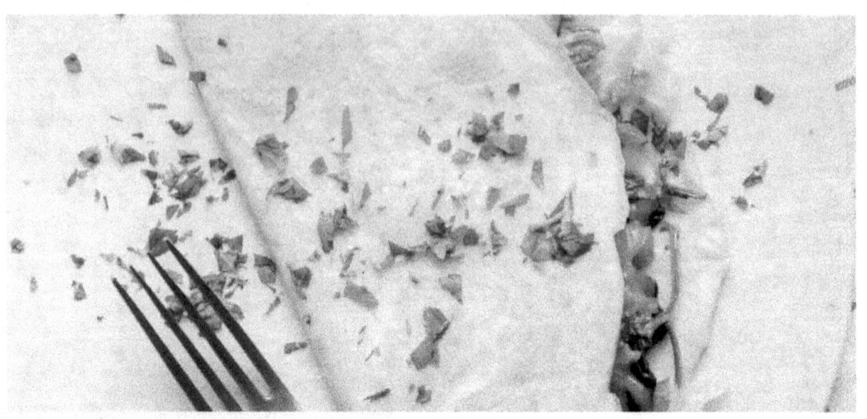

Veggie Omelette

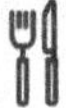 1 servings 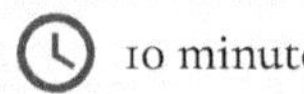 10 minutes

INGREDIENTS

2 eggs

1/4 cup chopped bell peppers (any color)

1/4 cup chopped onion

1/4 cup chopped spinach

1/4 cup shredded cheese

Salt and pepper to taste

1 teaspoon olive oil

NUTRITIONAL VALUE

300 calories,

20g protein,

20g fat,

10g carbohydrates,

3g fiber

DIRECTIONS

1. 1. In a bowl, beat the eggs with a fork and season with salt and pepper.
2. 2. Heat the olive oil in a non-stick skillet over medium heat.
3. 3. Add the bell peppers, onion, and spinach to the skillet and sauté for 2-3 minutes.
4. 4. Pour the beaten eggs over the vegetables and cook for 2-3 minutes, or until the eggs start to set.
5. 5. Sprinkle the shredded cheese over the eggs and fold the omelette in half.
6. 6. Cook for another minute, or until the cheese is melted.
7. 7. Serve hot and enjoy!

NOTES

This fluffy omelette is filled with colorful vegetables and melted cheese, making it a delicious and nutritious way to start your day.

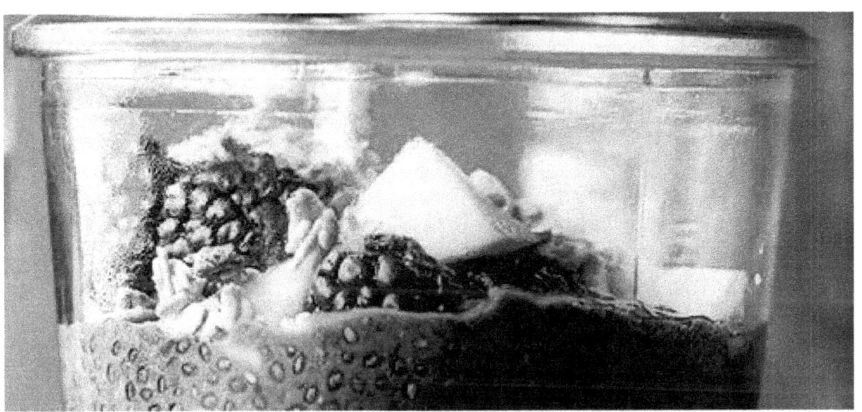

Chia Seed Pudding

DIRECTIONS

1. 2 tablespoons chia seeds
2. - 1/2 cup almond milk
3. - 1/4 teaspoon vanilla extract
4. - 1/2 cup mixed berries (strawberries, blueberries, raspberries)

🍴 1 servings   🕐 5 minutes

INGREDIENTS

2 tablespoons chia seeds

1/2 cup almond milk

1/4 teaspoon vanilla extract

1/2 cup mixed berries (strawberries, blueberries, raspberries)

NUTRITIONAL VALUE

200 calories,

5g protein,

10g fat,

20g carbohydrates,

10g fiber

NOTES

This chia seed pudding is made with almond milk and topped with fresh berries, making it a delicious and nutritious breakfast option.

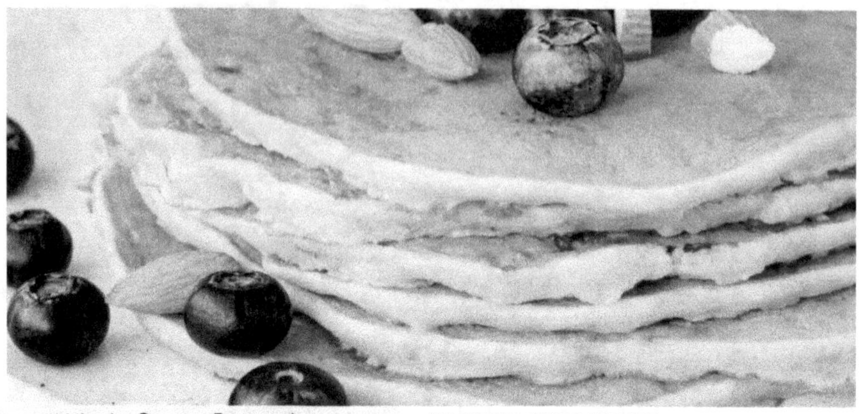

Whole Grain Pancakes

🍴 2 pancakes 🕐 15 minutes

INGREDIENTS

1/2 cup whole wheat flour

1/2 teaspoon baking powder

1/4 teaspoon baking soda

1/4 teaspoon salt

1/2 cup milk

1 tablespoon honey or maple syrup

1 egg

1 tablespoon melted butter or oil

Fresh fruit and maple syrup, for serving

NUTRITIONAL VALUE

250 calories,

8g protein,

5g fat,

45g carbohydrates,

5g fiber

DIRECTIONS

1.1. In a bowl, whisk together the whole wheat flour, baking powder, baking soda, and salt.

2.2. In another bowl, whisk together the milk, honey or maple syrup, egg, and melted butter or oil.

3.3. Pour the wet ingredients into the dry ingredients and stir until just combined.

4.4. Heat a non-stick skillet over medium heat and lightly grease with butter or oil.

5.5. Pour 1/4 cup of batter onto the skillet for each pancake.

6.6. Cook for 2-3 minutes, or until bubbles form on the surface of the pancake.

7.7. Flip and cook for another 1-2 minutes, or until golden brown.

8.8. Serve the pancakes topped with fresh fruit and a drizzle of maple syrup.

> **NOTES**
> These whole grain pancakes are made with whole wheat flour and topped with fresh fruit and a drizzle of maple syrup for a satisfying and nutritious breakfast.

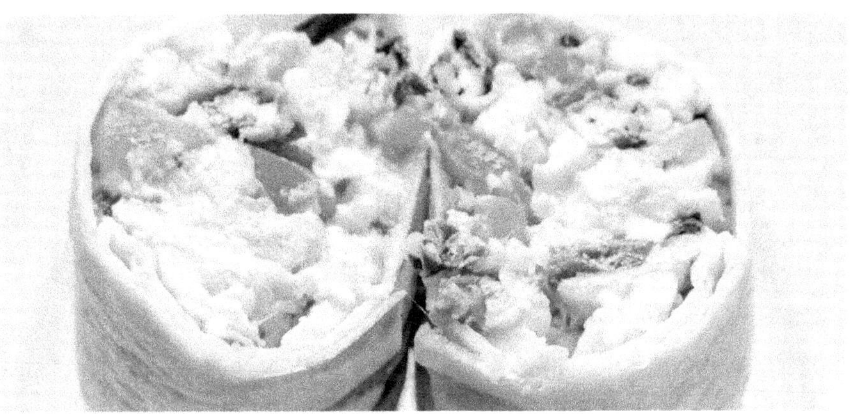

Breakfast Burrito

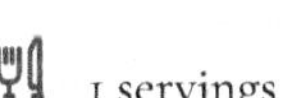 1 servings 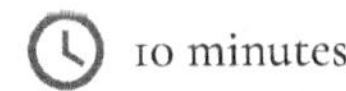 10 minutes

INGREDIENTS

2 eggs, scrambled

1/4 cup black beans, drained and rinsed

1/4 avocado, sliced

2 tablespoons salsa

1 whole grain tortilla

NUTRITIONAL VALUE

350 calories,

20g protein,

15g fat,

35g carbohydrates,

10g fiber

DIRECTIONS

1. 1. In a skillet, scramble the eggs until cooked through.
2. 2. Heat the black beans in the microwave or on the stove until warmed through.
3. 3. Heat the tortilla in the microwave or on the stove until warm and pliable.
4. 4. Place the scrambled eggs, black beans, avocado slices, and salsa in the center of the tortilla.
5. 5. Fold the sides of the tortilla over the filling and roll up tightly.
6. 6. Serve immediately and enjoy!

> **NOTES**
> This breakfast burrito is filled with scrambled eggs, black beans, avocado, and salsa, making it a satisfying and nutritious way to start your day.

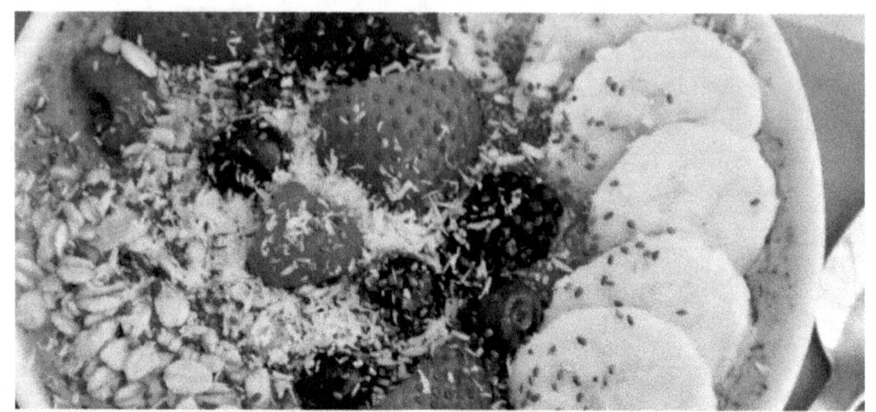

Smoothie Bowl

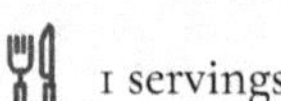 1 servings   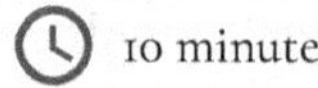 10 minutes

DIRECTIONS

1. 1. In a blender, combine the frozen banana, frozen berries, and almond milk.
2. 2. Blend until smooth and creamy.
3. 3. Pour the smoothie into a bowl.
4. 4. Top with chia seeds, granola, chopped nuts, and shredded coconut.
5. 5. Serve immediately and enjoy!

INGREDIENTS

1 frozen banana

1/2 cup frozen berries (any kind)

1/2 cup almond milk

1 tablespoon chia seeds

1 tablespoon granola

1 tablespoon chopped nuts
(almonds, walnuts, or pecans)

1 tablespoon shredded coconut

NUTRITIONAL VALUE

300 calories,

5g protein,

15g fat,

40g carbohydrates,

10g fiber

NOTES

This smoothie bowl is made with blended fruit and topped with granola, nuts, and seeds for a refreshing and nutritious breakfast.

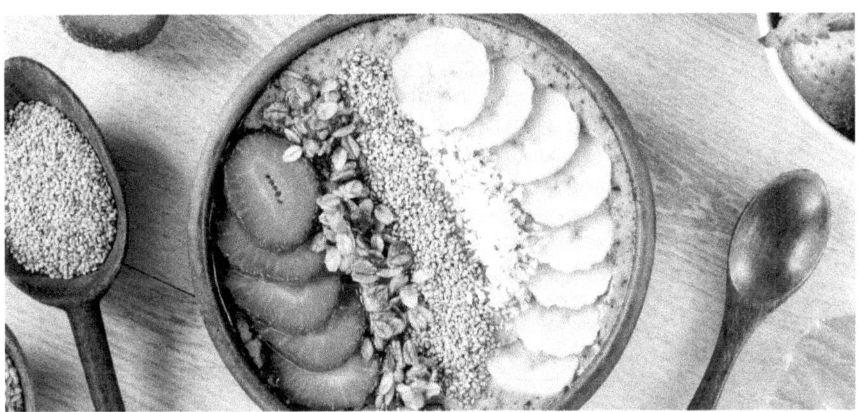

Breakfast Quinoa Bowl

DIRECTIONS

🍴 1 servings   🕐 10 minutes

INGREDIENTS

1/2 cup cooked quinoa

1/2 cup almond milk

1/4 teaspoon cinnamon

1 tablespoon chopped nuts (almonds, walnuts, or pecans)

1 tablespoon mixed seeds (chia seeds, flaxseeds, or hemp seeds)

1/4 cup mixed berries (strawberries, blueberries, raspberries)

NUTRITIONAL VALUE

300 calories,

10g protein,

10g fat,

40g carbohydrates,

8g fiber

1. 1. In a saucepan, heat the cooked quinoa with the almond milk and cinnamon until warmed through.
2. 2. Pour the quinoa mixture into a bowl.
3. 3. Top with chopped nuts, mixed seeds, and mixed berries.
4. 4. Serve immediately and enjoy!

NOTES

This breakfast quinoa bowl is made with cooked quinoa, almond milk, and topped with nuts, seeds, and fruit for a hearty and nutritious breakfast.

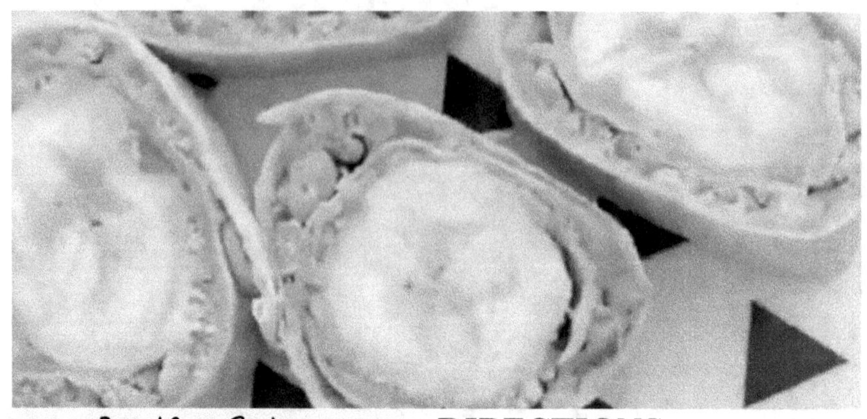

Breakfast Sushi

 1 servings  10 minutes

INGREDIENTS

1/2 cup rolled oats

1 cup water or milk

1 tablespoon almond butter

1/2 banana, sliced

1 teaspoon chia seeds

NUTRITIONAL VALUE

300 calories,

10g protein,

10g fat,

45g carbohydrates,

8g fiber

DIRECTIONS

1. 1. In a saucepan, bring the water or milk to a boil.
2. 2. Stir in the rolled oats and reduce heat to low.
3. 3. Cook for 5 minutes, stirring occasionally, until the oats are creamy.
4. 4. Spread the almond butter evenly over a sheet of parchment paper.
5. 5. Place the cooked oats on top of the almond butter.
6. 6. Place the banana slices along one edge of the oats.
7. 7. Roll up the oats and banana like a sushi roll.
8. 8. Slice the roll into bite-sized pieces.
9. 9. Sprinkle the chia seeds over the top.
10. 10. Serve immediately and enjoy!

NOTES
This breakfast sushi is made with rolled oats, almond butter, banana, and chia seeds, making it a fun and nutritious way to start your day.

25

VIBRANT SALAD

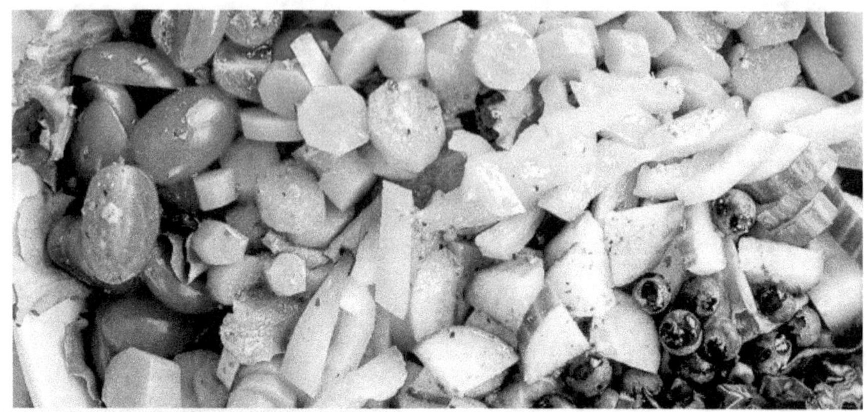

Rainbow Veggie Salad

DIRECTIONS

1. 1. In a large bowl, combine the mixed greens, cherry tomatoes, cucumber, bell peppers, red onion, olives, and feta cheese.
2. 2. In a small bowl, whisk together the olive oil, lemon juice, Dijon mustard, salt, and pepper.
3. 3. Pour the dressing over the salad and toss to combine.
4. 4. Serve immediately and enjoy!

2 servings　　🕐 15 minutes

INGREDIENTS

2 cups mixed greens

1/2 cup cherry tomatoes, halved

1/2 cup cucumber, diced

1/2 cup bell peppers, thinly sliced (any color)

1/4 cup red onion, thinly sliced

1/4 cup Kalamata olives, pitted

1/4 cup feta cheese, crumbled

2 tablespoons olive oil

1 tablespoon lemon juice

1 teaspoon Dijon mustard

Salt and pepper to taste

NUTRITIONAL VALUE

200 calories,

5g protein,

15g fat,

10g carbohydrates,

3g fiber

NOTES

This vibrant salad is packed with colorful vegetables and tossed in a zesty lemon vinaigrette, creating a refreshing and nutritious dish.

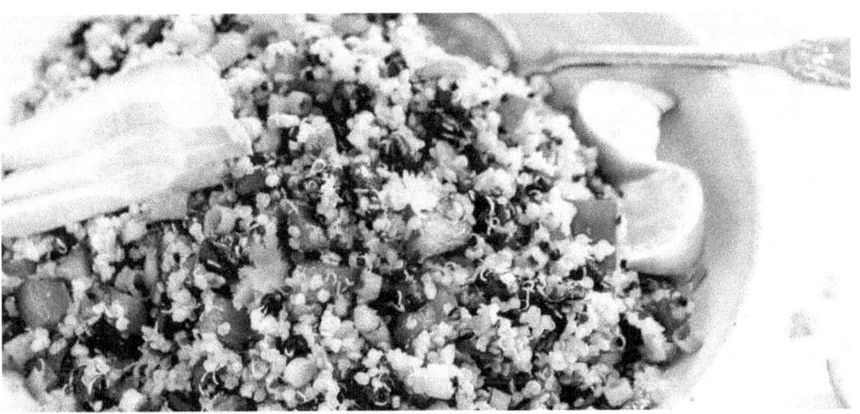

Quinoa and Black Bean Salad

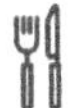 2 servings 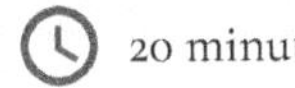 20 minutes

INGREDIENTS

1/2 cup quinoa

1 cup water or vegetable broth

1/2 cup black beans, drained and
rinsed

1/2 cup corn kernels (fresh or frozen)

1/2 avocado, diced

- 2 tablespoons fresh cilantro,
chopped

1 tablespoon olive oil

1 tablespoon lime juice

1/2 teaspoon cumin

Salt and pepper to taste

NUTRITIONAL VALUE

300 calories,

10g protein,

10g fat,

40g carbohydrates,

8g fiber

DIRECTIONS

1. 1. In a saucepan, combine the quinoa and water or broth.
2. 2. Bring to a boil, then reduce heat to low and simmer for 15 minutes, or until the quinoa is cooked and the liquid is absorbed.
3. 3. In a large bowl, combine the cooked quinoa, black beans, corn, avocado, and cilantro.
4. 4. In a small bowl, whisk together the olive oil, lime juice, cumin, salt, and pepper.
5. 5. Pour the dressing over the salad and toss to combine.
6. 6. Serve immediately and enjoy!

NOTES

This hearty salad is made with quinoa, black beans, corn, and avocado, tossed in a cilantro lime dressing for a fresh and flavorful dish.

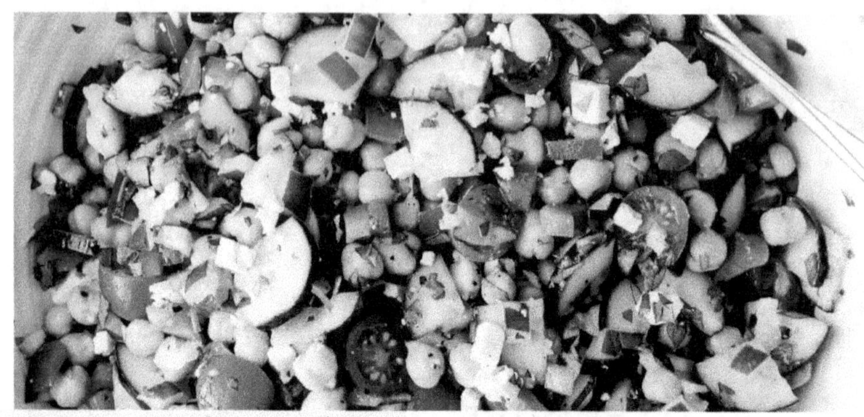

Mediterranean Chickpea Salad

🍴 2 servings   🕐 15 minutes

INGREDIENTS

1 can (15 oz) chickpeas, drained
and rinsed

1 cucumber, diced

1 cup cherry tomatoes, halved

1/4 cup red onion, thinly sliced

1/4 cup feta cheese, crumbled

2 tablespoons fresh parsley,
chopped

2 tablespoons olive oil

1 tablespoon lemon juice

1 teaspoon dried oregano

Salt and pepper to taste

NUTRITIONAL VALUE

250 calories,

10g protein,

10g fat,

30g carbohydrates,

8g fiber

DIRECTIONS

1. 1. In a large bowl, combine the chickpeas, cucumber, tomatoes, red onion, feta cheese, and parsley.
2. 2. In a small bowl, whisk together the olive oil, lemon juice, oregano, salt, and pepper.
3. 3. Pour the dressing over the salad and toss to combine.
4. 4. Serve immediately and enjoy!

NOTES

This Mediterranean-inspired salad is made with chickpeas, cucumber, tomatoes, red onion, and feta cheese, tossed in a lemon herb dressing for a refreshing and satisfying dish.

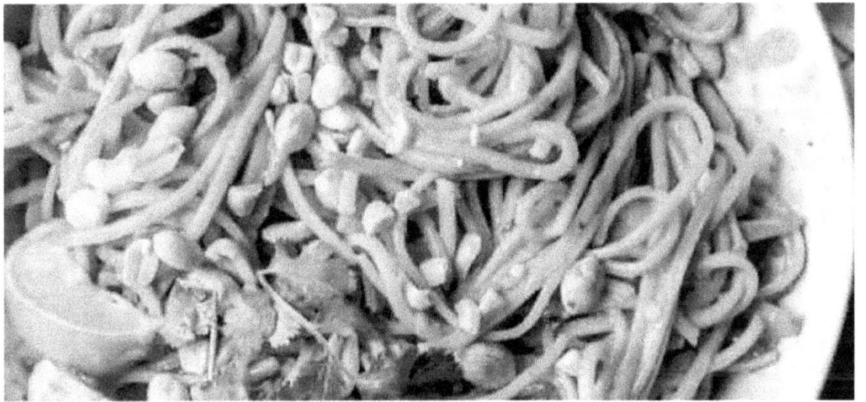

Asian-Inspired Noodle Salad

🍴 2 servings 🕐 20 minutes

INGREDIENTS

4 oz soba noodles

1 cup edamame, shelled

1/2 cup carrots, julienned

1/2 cup red bell pepper, thinly sliced

1 cup cabbage, thinly sliced

2 tablespoons sesame oil

2 tablespoons rice vinegar

1 tablespoon soy sauce

1 tablespoon honey

1 teaspoon fresh ginger, grated

1 clove garlic, minced

Sesame seeds for garnish

NUTRITIONAL VALUE

350 calories,

15g protein,

10g fat,

50g carbohydrates,

8g fiber

DIRECTIONS

1. 1. Cook the soba noodles according to package instructions, then rinse under cold water and drain.
2. 2. In a large bowl, combine the noodles, edamame, carrots, bell pepper, and cabbage.
3. 3. In a small bowl, whisk together the sesame oil, rice vinegar, soy sauce, honey, ginger, and garlic.
4. 4. Pour the dressing over the salad and toss to combine.
5. 5. Serve immediately, sprinkled with sesame seeds.

NOTES

This Asian-inspired salad is made with noodles, edamame, carrots, bell peppers, and cabbage, tossed in a sesame ginger dressing for a flavorful and satisfying dish.

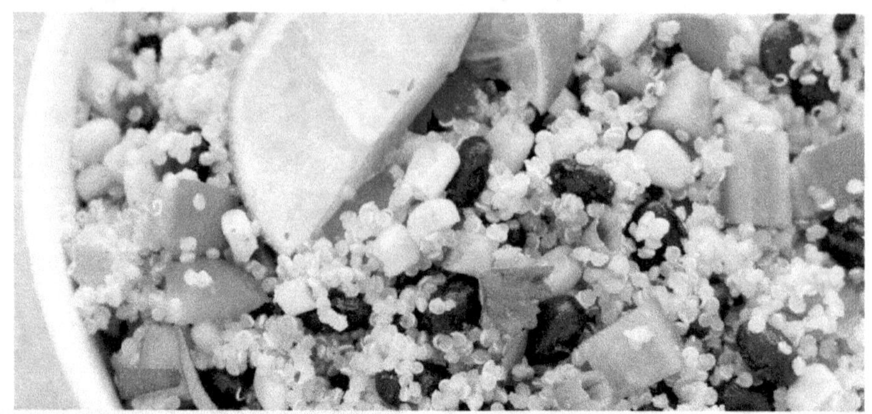

Southwest Quinoa Salad

 2 servings    20 minutes

INGREDIENTS

1/2 cup quinoa

1 cup water or vegetable broth

1/2 cup black beans, drained and rinsed

1/2 cup corn kernels (fresh or frozen)

1/2 cup bell peppers, diced (any color)

1/2 avocado, diced

2 tablespoons fresh cilantro, chopped

2 tablespoons olive oil

1 tablespoon lime juice

1/2 teaspoon chipotle powder

Salt and pepper to taste

NUTRITIONAL VALUE

300 calories,

10g protein,

10g fat,

40g carbohydrates,

8g fiber

DIRECTIONS

1. 1. In a saucepan, combine the quinoa and water or broth.

2. 2. Bring to a boil, then reduce heat to low and simmer for 15 minutes, or until the quinoa is cooked and the liquid is absorbed.

3. 3. In a large bowl, combine the cooked quinoa, black beans, corn, bell peppers, avocado, and cilantro.

4. 4. In a small bowl, whisk together the olive oil, lime juice, chipotle powder, salt, and pepper.

5. 5. Pour the dressing over the salad and toss to combine.

6. 6. Serve immediately and enjoy!

NOTES

This spicy salad is made with quinoa, black beans, corn, bell peppers, and avocado, tossed in a chipotle lime dressing for a flavorful and satisfying dish.

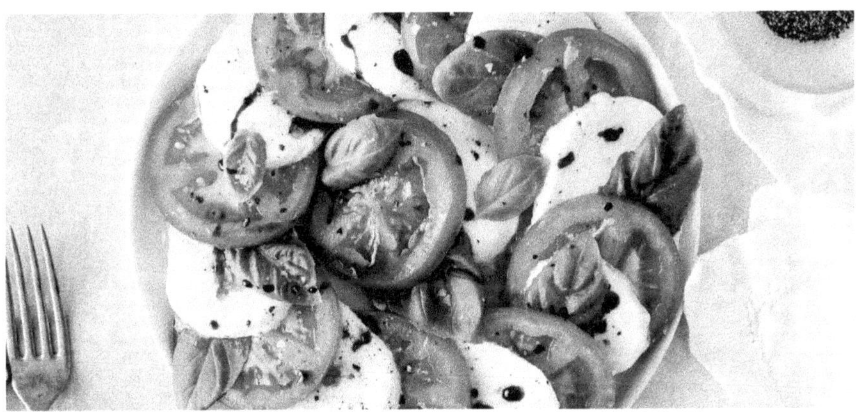

Caprese Salad

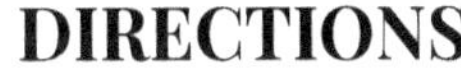

🍴 2 servings   🕐 10 minutes

INGREDIENTS

2 large tomatoes, sliced

1/2 cup fresh basil
leaves

4 oz fresh mozzarella
cheese, sliced

2 tablespoons balsamic
glaze

Salt and pepper to taste

NUTRITIONAL VALUE

250 calories,

15g protein,

15g fat,

10g carbohydrates,

3g fiber

DIRECTIONS

1.1. Arrange the tomato slices on a serving platter.

2.2. Top each tomato slice with a basil leaf and a slice of mozzarella cheese.

3.3. Drizzle the balsamic glaze over the salad.

4.4. Season with salt and pepper to taste.

5.5. Serve immediately and enjoy!

NOTES

This classic Italian salad is made with fresh tomatoes, basil, and mozzarella cheese, drizzled with balsamic glaze for a simple and delicious dish.

32

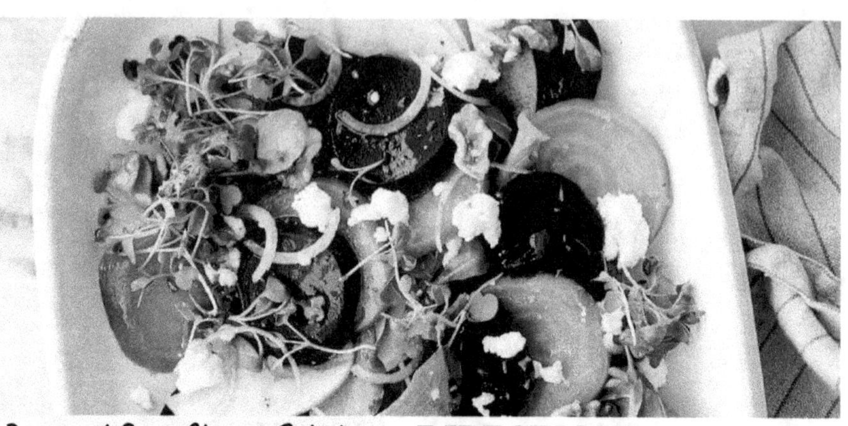

Beet and Goat Cheese Salad

🍴 2 servings   🕐 30 minutes

INGREDIENTS

2 medium beets, roasted
and peeled

2 cups mixed greens

1/4 cup goat cheese,
crumbled

1/4 cup walnuts, chopped

2 tablespoons olive oil

1 tablespoon balsamic
vinegar

1 teaspoon honey

Salt and pepper to taste

NUTRITIONAL VALUE

300 calories,

10g protein,

15g fat,

30g carbohydrates,

8g fiber

DIRECTIONS

1. 1. Preheat the oven to 400°F (200°C).

2. 2. Wrap the beets in foil and roast in the oven for 25-30 minutes, or until tender.

3. 3. Let the beets cool, then peel and slice them.

4. 4. In a large bowl, combine the mixed greens, roasted beets, goat cheese, and walnuts.

5. 5. In a small bowl, whisk together the olive oil, balsamic vinegar, honey, salt, and pepper.

6. 6. Pour the dressing over the salad and toss to combine.

7. 7. Serve immediately and enjoy!

NOTES

This salad is made with roasted beets, creamy goat cheese, and crunchy walnuts, tossed in a balsamic vinaigrette for a flavorful and satisfying dish.

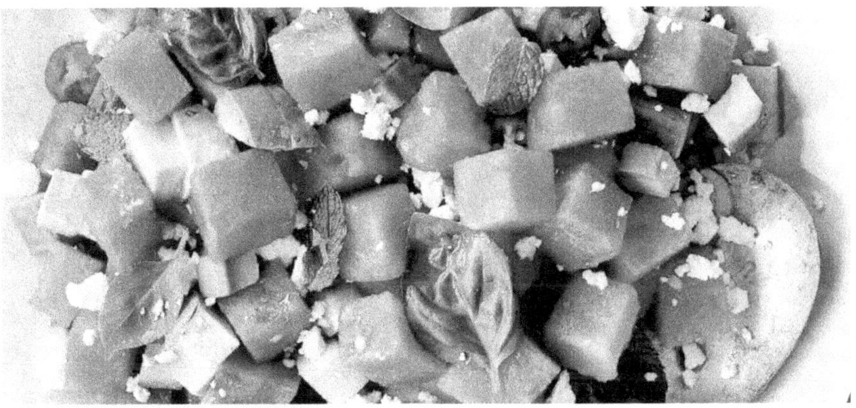

Watermelon and Feta Salad

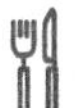 2 servings   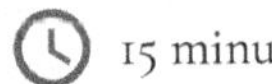 15 minutes

INGREDIENTS

2 cups cubed watermelon

1/2 cup crumbled feta

cheese

2 tablespoons fresh mint,

chopped

1 tablespoon olive oil

1 tablespoon lime juice

Salt and pepper to taste

NUTRITIONAL VALUE

200 calories,

5g protein,

10g fat,

20g carbohydrates,

3g fiber

DIRECTIONS

1. 1. In a large bowl, combine the watermelon, feta cheese, and mint.
2. 2. In a small bowl, whisk together the olive oil, lime juice, salt, and pepper.
3. 3. Pour the dressing over the salad and toss to combine.
4. 4. Serve immediately and enjoy!

NOTES

This refreshing salad is made with juicy watermelon, creamy feta cheese, and fresh mint, tossed in a lime dressing for a light and flavorful dish.

34

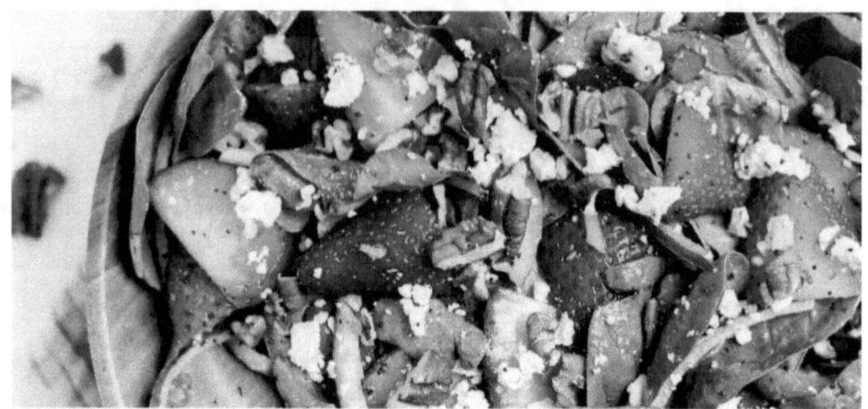

Spinach and Strawberry Salad

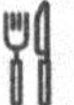 2 servings  15 minutes

INGREDIENTS

2 cups fresh spinach leaves

1 cup sliced strawberries

1/4 cup sliced almonds

1/4 cup crumbled feta
cheese

2 tablespoons olive oil

1 tablespoon balsamic
vinegar

1 teaspoon honey

Salt and pepper to taste

NUTRITIONAL VALUE

250 calories,

8g protein,

15g fat,

25g carbohydrates,

5g fiber

DIRECTIONS

1. 1. In a large bowl, combine the spinach, strawberries, almonds, and feta cheese.
2. 2. In a small bowl, whisk together the olive oil, balsamic vinegar, honey, salt, and pepper.
3. 3. Pour the dressing over the salad and toss to combine.
4. 4. Serve immediately and enjoy!

NOTES

This salad is made with fresh spinach, sweet strawberries, crunchy almonds, and tangy feta cheese, tossed in a balsamic vinaigrette for a delicious and nutritious dish.

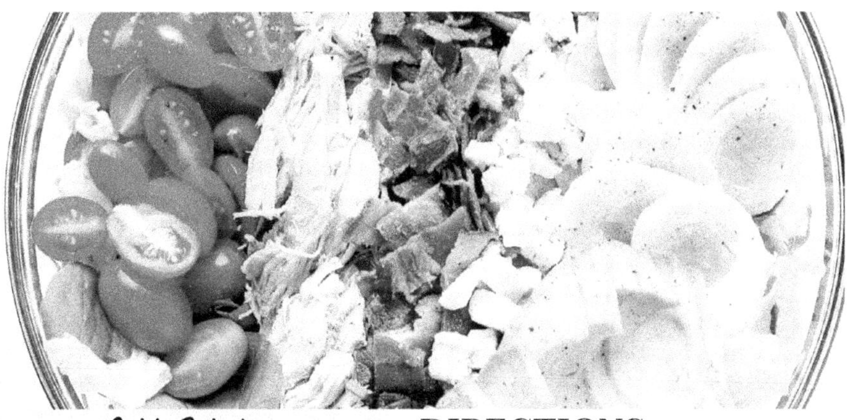

Cobb Salad

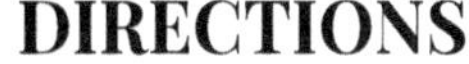 2 servings 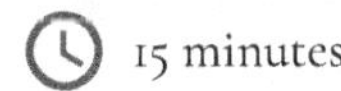 15 minutes

DIRECTIONS

1. Mix all the ingredients together, excluding the dressing, salt, and pepper, in a big bowl or on a serving platter.
2. Toss to mix in the dressing.
3. Use salt and pepper to season to taste.

INGREDIENTS

2 cups Romaine lettuce

3 cups Watercress

5 slices Cooked bacon

6 oz Cooked chicken breast

1 cups Grape tomatoes

1 medium Avocados

1 large eggs

NUTRITIONAL VALUE

428 calories,

24.7g protein,

33.5g fat,

25g carbohydrates,

4.6g fiber

NOTES

This recipe combines creamy avocado with a perfectly poached egg on top of crunchy whole grain toast, creating a satisfying and nutritious breakfast.

Hearty soups

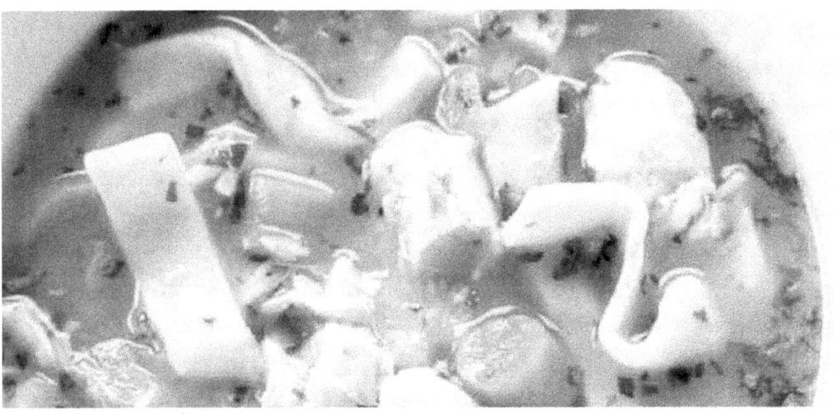

Chicken Noodle Soup

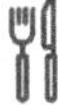 4 servings 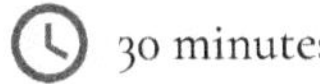 30 minutes

INGREDIENTS

1 tablespoon olive oil

1 onion, chopped

2 carrots, sliced

2 celery stalks, sliced

2 garlic cloves, minced

6 cups chicken broth

2 cups shredded cooked chicken

2 cups egg noodles

1 teaspoon dried thyme

Salt and pepper to taste

Fresh parsley for garnish

NUTRITIONAL VALUE

300 calories,

20g protein,

10g fat,

30g carbohydrates,

3g fiber

DIRECTIONS

1. 1. In a large pot, heat the olive oil over medium heat.
2. 2. Add the onion, carrots, celery, and garlic. Cook until vegetables are softened, about 5 minutes.
3. 3. Add the chicken broth, chicken, noodles, and thyme. Bring to a boil.
4. 4. Reduce heat and simmer until noodles are tender, about 10 minutes.
5. 5. Season with salt and pepper.
6. 6. Serve hot, garnished with fresh parsley.

NOTES

This classic soup is made with tender chicken, hearty vegetables, and egg noodles in a flavorful broth, perfect for warming up on a chilly day.

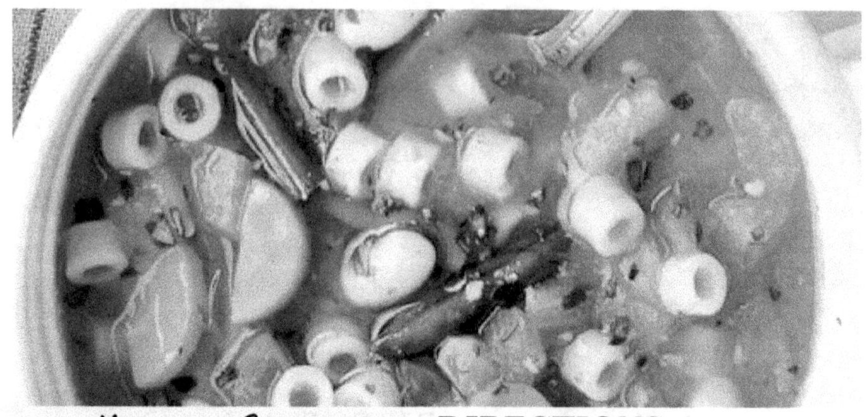

Minestrone Soup

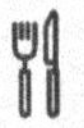 4 servings 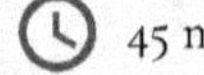 45 minutes

INGREDIENTS

tablespoon olive oil

1 onion, chopped

2 carrots, diced

2 celery stalks, diced

2 garlic cloves, minced

1 can (15 oz) diced tomatoes

4 cups vegetable broth

1 can (15 oz) kidney beans, drained and rinsed

1 cup small pasta (such as ditalini or small shells)

1 teaspoon dried basil

1 teaspoon dried oregano

Salt and pepper to taste

Grated Parmesan cheese for serving

NUTRITIONAL VALUE

250 calories,

10g protein,

5g fat,

40g carbohydrates,

8g fiber

DIRECTIONS

1. 1. In a large pot, heat the olive oil over medium heat.

2. 2. Add the onion, carrots, celery, and garlic. Cook until vegetables are softened, about 5 minutes.

3. 3. Add the diced tomatoes, vegetable broth, kidney beans, pasta, basil, and oregano. Bring to a boil.

4. 4. Reduce heat and simmer until pasta is tender, about 15 minutes.

5. 5. Season with salt and pepper.

6. 6. Serve hot, topped with grated Parmesan cheese.

NOTES

This hearty soup is made with a variety of vegetables, beans, and pasta in a savory tomato broth, perfect for a satisfying and nutritious meal.

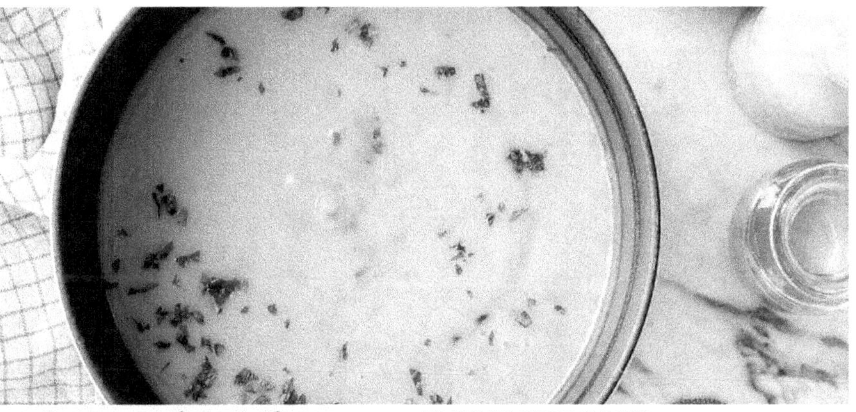

Butternut Squash Soup

 4 servings  1 hour

INGREDIENTS

1 butternut squash, peeled,
seeded, and diced

1 onion, chopped

2 garlic cloves, minced

4 cups vegetable broth

1 teaspoon ground cumin

1/2 teaspoon ground cinnamon

1/4 teaspoon ground nutmeg

Salt and pepper to taste

Coconut milk for serving

NUTRITIONAL VALUE

200 calories,

5g protein,

5g fat,

30g carbohydrates,

5g fiber

DIRECTIONS

1. 1. Preheat the oven to 400°F (200°C).
2. 2. Place the diced butternut squash on a baking sheet lined with parchment paper.
3. 3. Roast in the oven for 30-40 minutes, or until tender and lightly browned.
4. 4. In a large pot, heat some olive oil over medium heat.
5. 5. Add the onion and garlic. Cook until softened, about 5 minutes.
6. 6. Add the roasted butternut squash, vegetable broth, cumin, cinnamon, nutmeg, salt, and pepper. Bring to a boil.
7. 7. Reduce heat and simmer for 10-15 minutes.
8. 8. Use an immersion blender to blend the soup until smooth.
9. 9. Serve hot, drizzled with coconut milk.

NOTES

This creamy soup is made with roasted butternut squash, onions, and warming spices, blended to perfection for a comforting and delicious dish.

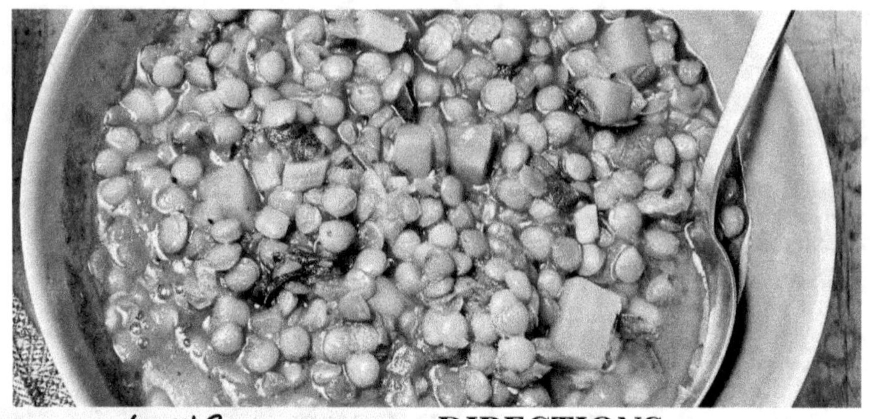

Lentil Soup

🍴 4 servings   🕐 45 minutes

INGREDIENTS

1 tablespoon olive oil

1 onion, chopped

2 carrots, diced

2 celery stalks, diced

2 garlic cloves, minced

1 cup dried green or brown lentils, rinsed

4 cups vegetable broth

1 can (15 oz) diced tomatoes

1 teaspoon ground cumin

1/2 teaspoon ground coriander

1/4 teaspoon cayenne pepper

Salt and pepper to taste

Fresh cilantro for serving

NUTRITIONAL VALUE

250 calories,

15g protein,

5g fat,

40g carbohydrates,

10g fiber

DIRECTIONS

1. 1. In a large pot, heat the olive oil over medium heat.

2. 2. Add the onion, carrots, celery, and garlic. Cook until vegetables are softened, about 5 minutes.

3. 3. Add the lentils, vegetable broth, diced tomatoes, cumin, coriander, cayenne pepper, salt, and pepper. Bring to a boil.

4. 4. Reduce heat and simmer until lentils are tender, about 30-40 minutes.

5. 5. Serve hot, garnished with fresh cilantro.

NOTES

This hearty soup is made with lentils, vegetables, and warming spices, perfect for a nutritious and satisfying meal.

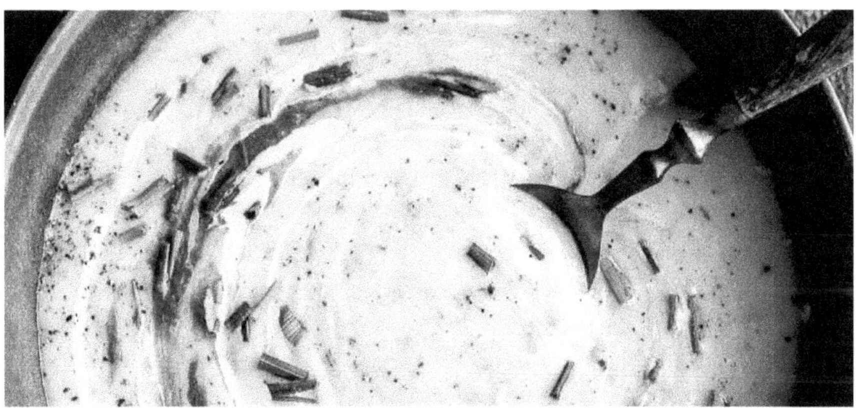

Potato Leek Soup

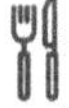 4 servings 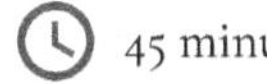 45 minutes

INGREDIENTS

2 tablespoons olive oil

2 leeks, white and light green
parts only, sliced

2 garlic cloves, minced

4 cups vegetable broth

4 cups potatoes, peeled and diced

1/2 cup heavy cream

Salt and pepper to taste

Chives for garnish

NUTRITIONAL VALUE

300 calories,

5g protein,

15g fat,

40g carbohydrates,

5g fiber

DIRECTIONS

1. 1. In a large pot, heat the olive oil over medium heat.

2. 2. Add the leeks and garlic. Cook until softened, about 5 minutes.

3. 3. Add the vegetable broth and potatoes. Bring to a boil.

4. 4. Reduce heat and simmer until potatoes are tender, about 20–25 minutes.

5. 5. Use an immersion blender to blend the soup until smooth.

6. 6. Stir in the heavy cream.

7. 7. Season with salt and pepper.

8. 8. Serve hot, garnished with chives.

NOTES

This creamy soup is made with potatoes, leeks, and garlic, blended to perfection for a velvety texture and rich flavor.

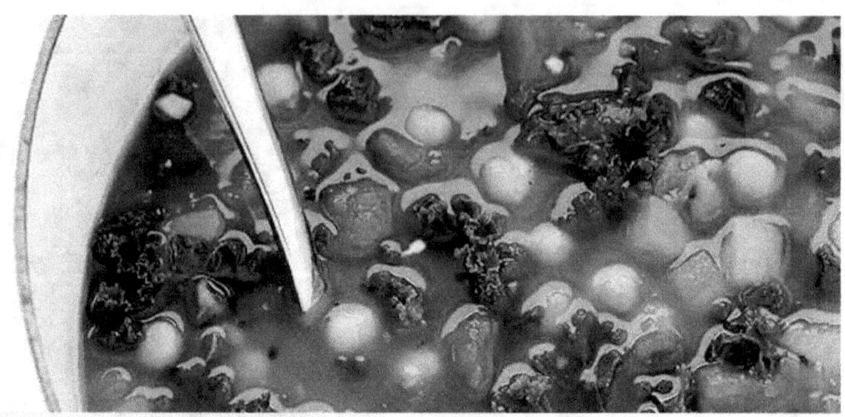

Moroccan Chickpea Soup

 4 servings  45 minutes

INGREDIENTS

1 tablespoon olive oil

1 onion, chopped

2 carrots, diced

2 celery stalks, diced

2 garlic cloves, minced

1 teaspoon ground cumin

1 teaspoon ground coriander

1/2 teaspoon ground cinnamon

1/4 teaspoon cayenne pepper

1 can (15 oz) chickpeas, drained and rinsed

1 can (15 oz) diced tomatoes

4 cups vegetable broth

Salt and pepper to taste

Fresh cilantro for serving

NUTRITIONAL VALUE

250 calories,

10g protein,

5g fat,

40g carbohydrates,

10g fiber

DIRECTIONS

1.1. In a large pot, heat the olive oil over medium heat.

2.2. Add the onion, carrots, celery, and garlic. Cook until vegetables are softened, about 5 minutes.

3.3. Add the cumin, coriander, cinnamon, and cayenne pepper. Cook for another minute, until fragrant.

4.4. Add the chickpeas, diced tomatoes, and vegetable broth. Bring to a boil.

5.5. Reduce heat and simmer for 20-30 minutes.

6.6. Season with salt and pepper.

7.7. Serve hot, garnished with fresh cilantro.

NOTES

This spicy soup is made with chickpeas, tomatoes, and warming spices, perfect for a flavorful and satisfying meal.

43

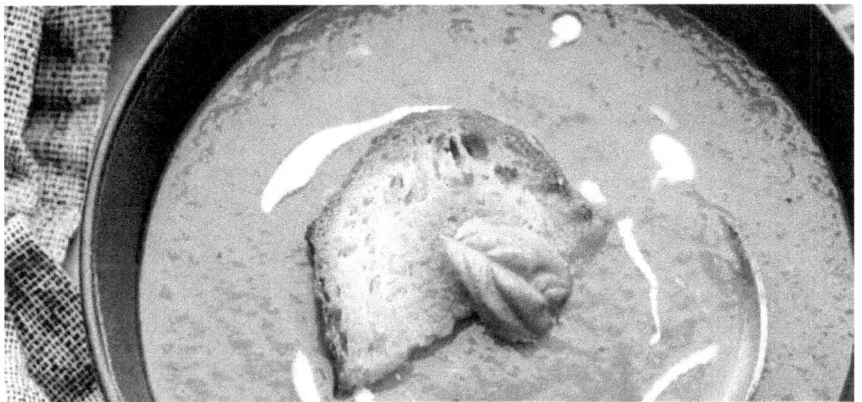

Tomato Basil Soup

 4 servings  30

INGREDIENTS

1 tablespoon olive oil

1 onion, chopped

2 garlic cloves, minced

2 cans (15 oz each) diced tomatoes

4 cups vegetable broth

1/4 cup fresh basil leaves, chopped

Salt and pepper to taste

Grated Parmesan cheese for serving

NUTRITIONAL VALUE

200 calories,

5g protein,

5g fat,

30g carbohydrates,

5g fiber

DIRECTIONS

1.1. In a large pot, heat the olive oil over medium heat.

2.2. Add the onion and garlic. Cook until softened, about 5 minutes.

3.3. Add the diced tomatoes (with their juices) and vegetable broth. Bring to a boil.

4.4. Reduce heat and simmer for 15-20 minutes.

5.5. Use an immersion blender to blend the soup until smooth.

6.6. Stir in the chopped basil.

7.7. Season with salt and pepper.

8.8. Serve hot, topped with grated Parmesan cheese.

NOTES

This classic soup is made with tomatoes, basil, and garlic, blended to perfection for a velvety texture and rich flavor.

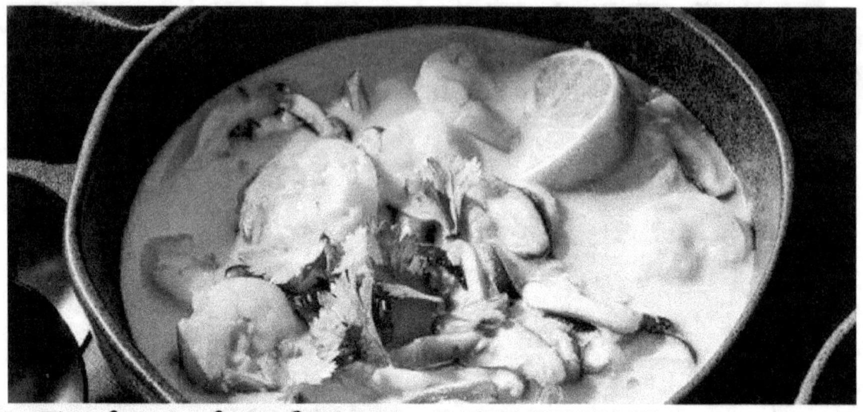

Thai Coconut Curry Soup

 4 servings   🕐 45 minutes

INGREDIENTS

1 tablespoon olive oil

1 onion, chopped

2 garlic cloves, minced

1 tablespoon Thai red curry paste

4 cups vegetable broth

1 can (14 oz) coconut milk

1 tablespoon soy sauce

1 tablespoon brown sugar

2 cups mixed vegetables (such as bell peppers, broccoli, and carrots)

1 block tofu, cubed

Fresh cilantro for serving

NUTRITIONAL VALUE

300 calories,

10g protein,

20g fat,

20g carbohydrates,

5g fiber

DIRECTIONS

1. 1. In a large pot, heat the olive oil over medium heat.
2. 2. Add the onion and garlic. Cook until softened, about 5 minutes.
3. 3. Add the curry paste. Cook for another minute, until fragrant.
4. 4. Add the vegetable broth, coconut milk, soy sauce, and brown sugar. Bring to a boil.
5. 5. Reduce heat and simmer for 10 minutes.
6. 6. Add the mixed vegetables and tofu. Simmer for another 10 minutes, or until vegetables are tender.
7. 7. Serve hot, garnished with fresh cilantro.

NOTES

This spicy soup is made with coconut milk, curry paste, vegetables, and tofu, perfect for a satisfying and exotic meal.

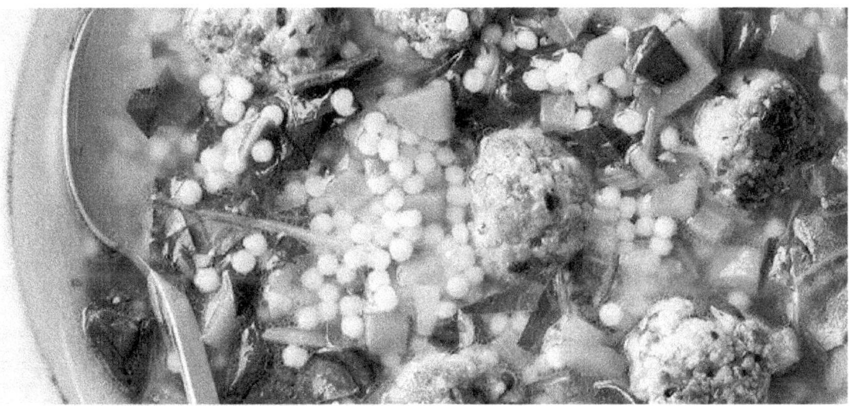

Italian Wedding Soup

 4 servings   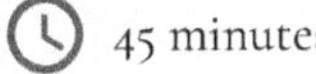 45 minutes

INGREDIENTS

1 tablespoon olive oil

1 onion, chopped

2 carrots, diced

2 celery stalks, diced

2 garlic cloves, minced

4 cups chicken broth

1/2 lb ground chicken

1/4 cup breadcrumbs

- 1 egg

1/4 cup grated Parmesan cheese

1/2 cup small pasta (such as orzo or acini di pepe)

2 cups baby spinach

Salt and pepper to taste

NUTRITIONAL VALUE

300 calories,

15g protein,

10g fat,

40g carbohydrates,

5g fiber

DIRECTIONS

1. 1. In a large pot, heat the olive oil over medium heat.

2. 2. Add the onion, carrots, celery, and garlic. Cook until vegetables are softened, about 5 minutes.

3. 3. Add the chicken broth. Bring to a boil.

4. 4. In a bowl, combine the ground chicken, breadcrumbs, egg, Parmesan cheese, salt, and pepper. Form into small meatballs.

5. 5. Drop the meatballs into the boiling broth. Cook for 5 minutes.

6. 6. Add the pasta and cook according to package instructions.

7. 7. Stir in the baby spinach and cook until wilted.

8. 8. Serve hot.

NOTES

This classic soup is made with meatballs, vegetables, and pasta in a savory broth, perfect for a comforting and satisfying meal.

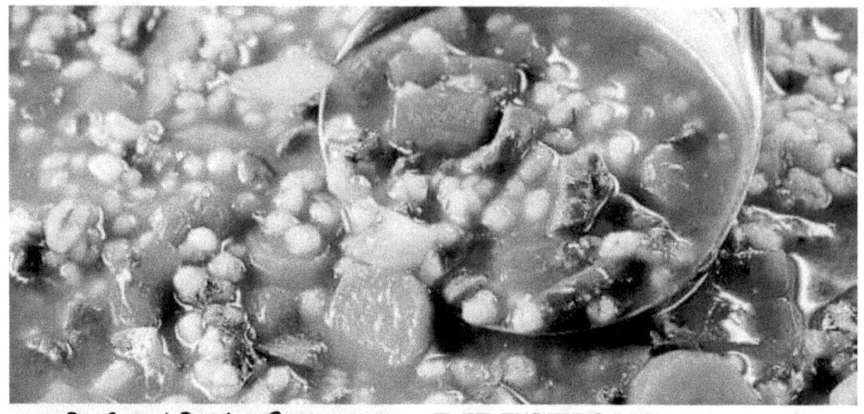

Beef and Barley Soup

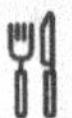 4 servings 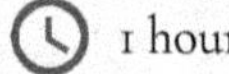 1 hour

INGREDIENTS

1 tablespoon olive oil

1 onion, chopped

2 carrots, diced

2 celery stalks, diced

2 garlic cloves, minced

1 lb beef stew meat, cubed

4 cups beef broth

1/2 cup pearl barley

1 teaspoon dried thyme

1 teaspoon dried rosemary

Salt and pepper to taste

Fresh parsley for serving

DIRECTIONS

1. 1. In a large pot, heat the olive oil over medium heat.
2. 2. Add the onion, carrots, celery, and garlic. Cook until vegetables are softened, about 5 minutes.
3. 3. Add the beef stew meat. Cook until browned on all sides.
4. 4. Add the beef broth, barley, thyme, rosemary, salt, and pepper. Bring to a boil.
5. 5. Reduce heat and simmer for 45–60 minutes, or until beef and barley are tender.
6. 6. Serve hot, garnished with fresh parsley.

NUTRITIONAL VALUE

350 calories,

20g protein,

15g fat,

40g carbohydrates,

8g fiber

NOTES

This hearty soup is made with tender beef, barley, vegetables, and warming spices, perfect for a satisfying and nutritious meal.

Satisfying Mains

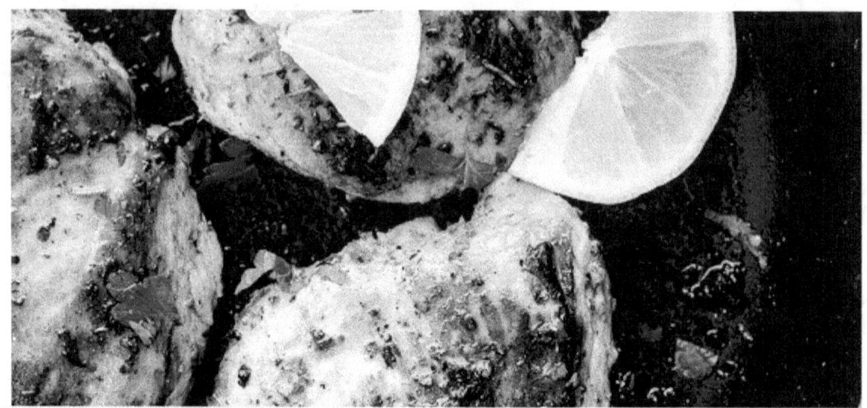

Lemon Herb Chicken

 4 servings  1 hour

INGREDIENTS

4 boneless, skinless chicken breasts

1/4 cup olive oil

2 tablespoons lemon juice

1 tablespoon fresh parsley, chopped

1 tablespoon fresh basil, chopped

1 tablespoon fresh thyme, chopped

2 garlic cloves, minced

Salt and pepper to taste

Lemon slices for garnish

NUTRITIONAL VALUE

250 calories,

30g protein,

10g fat,

5g carbohydrates,

1g fiber

DIRECTIONS

1. 1. In a small bowl, whisk together the olive oil, lemon juice, parsley, basil, thyme, garlic, salt, and pepper.
2. 2. Place the chicken breasts in a shallow dish and pour the marinade over them. Cover and refrigerate for at least 30 minutes, up to 4 hours.
3. 3. Preheat grill or oven to 375°F (190°C).
4. 4. Grill or bake the chicken for 25-30 minutes, or until cooked through, turning halfway through cooking.
5. 5. Serve hot, garnished with lemon slices.

NOTES

This succulent chicken is marinated in a zesty lemon herb mixture, then grilled or baked to perfection for a satisfying and flavorful main course.

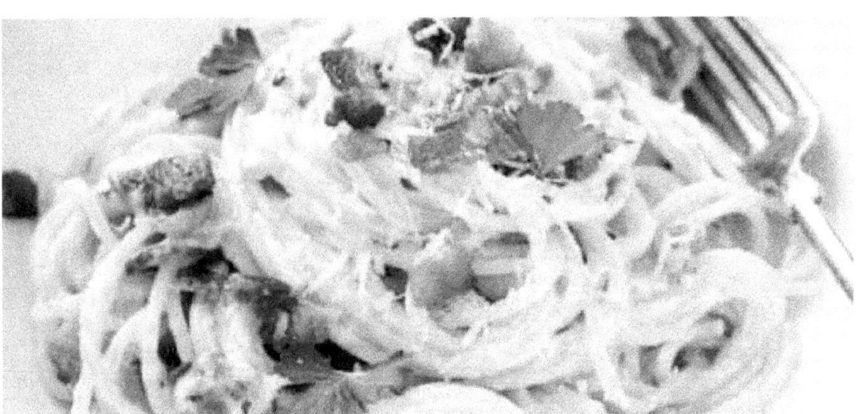

Spaghetti Carbonara

 4 servings  30 minutes

INGREDIENTS

12 oz spaghetti

4 oz pancetta, diced

2 garlic cloves, minced

2 eggs

1/2 cup grated Parmesan cheese

1/2 cup grated Pecorino Romano cheese

Salt and pepper to taste

Fresh parsley for garnish

NUTRITIONAL VALUE

400 calories,

20g protein,

15g fat,

50g carbohydrates,

3g fiber

DIRECTIONS

1.1. Cook the spaghetti according to package instructions. Drain, reserving 1/2 cup of pasta water.

2.2. In a large skillet, cook the pancetta over medium heat until crispy. Add the garlic and cook for another minute.

3.3. In a bowl, whisk together the eggs, Parmesan cheese, Pecorino Romano cheese, salt, and pepper.

4.4. Add the cooked spaghetti to the skillet with the pancetta and garlic. Remove from heat and quickly stir in the egg mixture, adding reserved pasta water as needed to create a creamy sauce.

5.5. Serve hot, garnished with fresh parsley.

> **NOTES**
> This classic Italian dish is made with spaghetti, pancetta, eggs, and cheese, creating a rich and creamy sauce that is sure to satisfy.

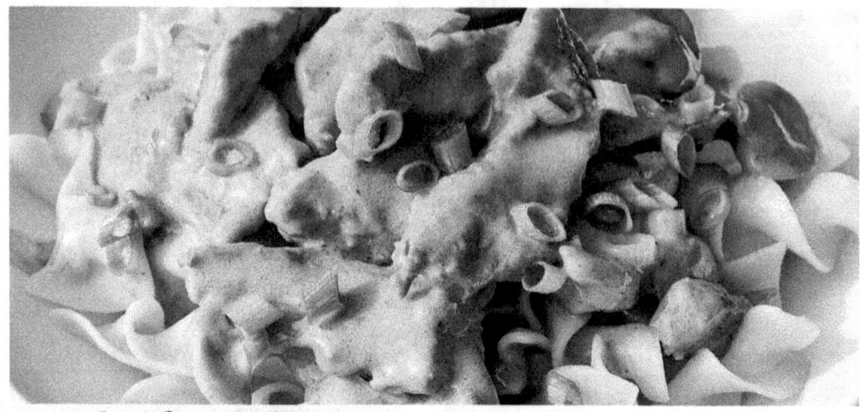

Beef Stroganoff

 4 servings    45 minutes

INGREDIENTS

1 lb beef sirloin, thinly sliced

1 onion, thinly sliced

8 oz mushrooms, sliced

2 garlic cloves, minced

1/2 cup beef broth

1 cup sour cream

1 tablespoon Dijon mustard

1 tablespoon Worcestershire sauce

Salt and pepper to taste

Fresh parsley for garnish

Cooked egg noodles for serving

NUTRITIONAL VALUE

400 calories,

30g protein,

20g fat,

30g carbohydrates,

3g fiber

DIRECTIONS

1. 1. In a large skillet, heat some olive oil over medium-high heat. Add the beef and cook until browned. Remove from skillet and set aside.

2. 2. In the same skillet, add a bit more olive oil if needed. Add the onion and mushrooms. Cook until softened, about 5 minutes.

3. 3. Add the garlic and cook for another minute.

4. 4. Return the beef to the skillet. Add the beef broth, sour cream, Dijon mustard, Worcestershire sauce, salt, and pepper. Stir to combine.

5. 5. Simmer for 10-15 minutes, until the sauce has thickened and the beef is cooked through.

6. 6. Serve hot over cooked egg noodles, garnished with fresh parsley.

NOTES

This classic dish is made with tender beef, mushrooms, and onions in a creamy sauce, served over egg noodles for a comforting and satisfying meal.

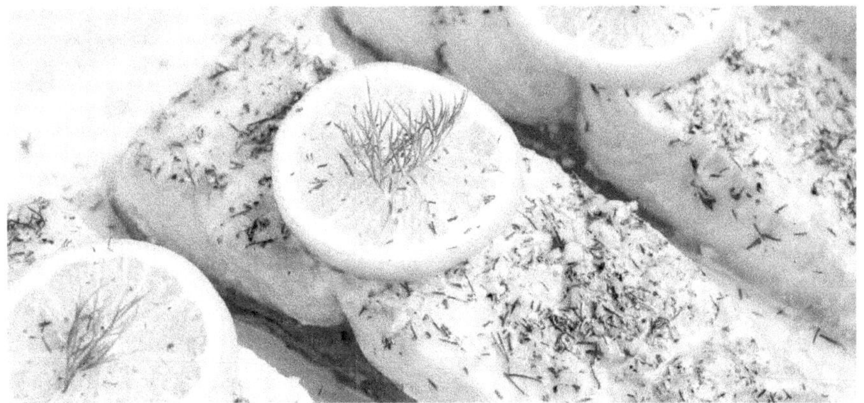

Baked Salmon with Lemon and Dill

 4 servings 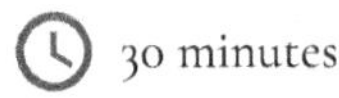 30 minutes

INGREDIENTS

4 salmon fillets

1/4 cup olive oil

2 tablespoons lemon juice

2 tablespoons fresh dill, chopped

2 garlic cloves, minced

Salt and pepper to taste

Lemon slices for garnish

NUTRITIONAL VALUE

300 calories,

30g protein,

15g fat,

5g carbohydrates,

1g fiber

DIRECTIONS

1. 1. Preheat oven to 375°F (190°C).

2. 2. In a small bowl, whisk together the olive oil, lemon juice, dill, garlic, salt, and pepper.

3. 3. Place the salmon fillets in a baking dish and pour the marinade over them. Cover and refrigerate for at least 30 minutes.

4. 4. Bake the salmon for 15-20 minutes, or until cooked through.

5. 5. Serve hot, garnished with lemon slices.

NOTES

This baked salmon is marinated in a mixture of lemon juice, dill, and garlic, then baked to perfection for a light and flavorful main course.

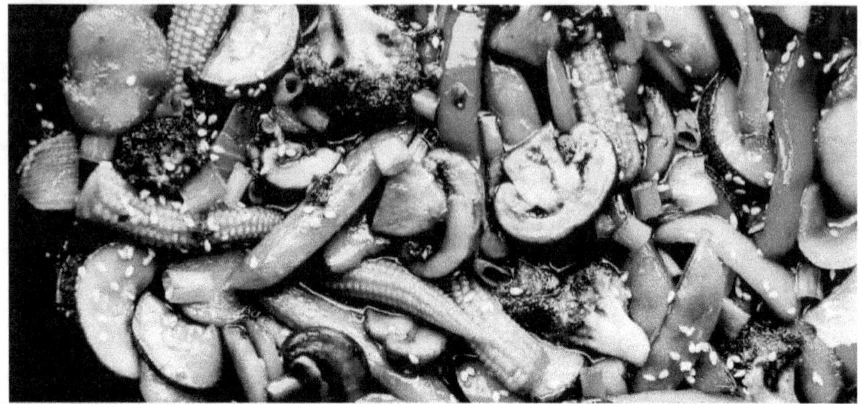

Vegetable Stir-Fry

 4 servings  30 minutes

INGREDIENTS

1 tablespoon olive oil

1 onion, sliced

2 bell peppers, sliced

2 carrots, sliced

1 zucchini, sliced

1 cup broccoli florets

1 cup snap peas

1 block tofu, cubed

1/4 cup soy sauce

2 tablespoons hoisin sauce

1 tablespoon sesame oil

1 tablespoon rice vinegar

1 tablespoon honey

2 garlic cloves, minced

1 teaspoon ginger, minced

Cooked rice for serving

NUTRITIONAL VALUE

300 calories,

15g protein,

10g fat,

40g carbohydrates,

8g fiber

DIRECTIONS

1. 1. In a large skillet or wok, heat the olive oil over medium-high heat.

2. 2. Add the onion, bell peppers, carrots, zucchini, broccoli, and snap peas. Stir-fry for 5-7 minutes, or until vegetables are tender-crisp.

3. 3. Add the tofu and cook for another 2-3 minutes.

4. 4. In a small bowl, whisk together the soy sauce, hoisin sauce, sesame oil, rice vinegar, honey, garlic, and ginger.

5. 5. Pour the sauce over the vegetables and tofu. Stir to combine and cook for another minute.

6. 6. Serve hot over cooked rice.

> **NOTES**
> This vibrant stir-fry is made with a variety of fresh vegetables, tofu, and a flavorful sauce, perfect for a nutritious and delicious meal.

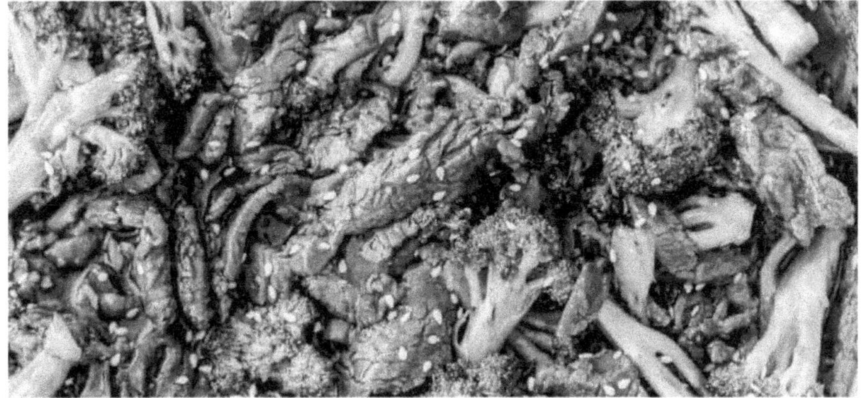

Beef and Broccoli Stir-Fry

 4 servings   🕒 30 minutes

INGREDIENTS

1 lb flank steak, thinly sliced

1/4 cup soy sauce

2 tablespoons oyster sauce

1 tablespoon hoisin sauce

1 tablespoon sesame oil

2 garlic cloves, minced

1 teaspoon ginger, minced

2 tablespoons olive oil

1 onion, sliced

2 cups broccoli florets

Cooked rice for serving

NUTRITIONAL VALUE

350 calories,

25g protein,

15g fat,

30g carbohydrates,

5g fiber

DIRECTIONS

1. 1. In a bowl, combine the soy sauce, oyster sauce, hoisin sauce, sesame oil, garlic, and ginger. Add the sliced beef and marinate for at least 15 minutes.

2. 2. In a large skillet or wok, heat the olive oil over medium-high heat.

3. 3. Add the onion and cook until softened, about 5 minutes.

4. 4. Add the marinated beef and cook for 3-4 minutes, or until browned.

5. 5. Add the broccoli florets and cook for another 3-4 minutes, or until tender-crisp.

6. 6. Serve hot over cooked rice.

> **NOTES**
> This classic stir-fry is made with tender beef, broccoli, and a savory sauce, perfect for a quick and delicious meal.

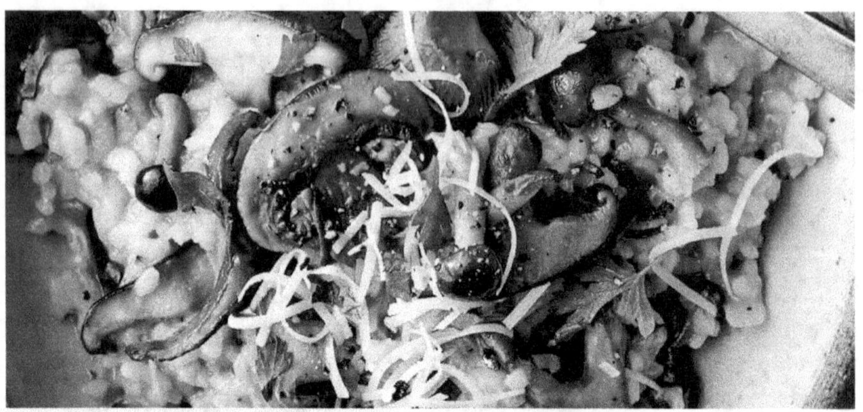

Mushroom Risotto

 4 servings 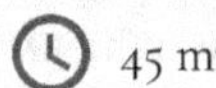 45 minutes

INGREDIENTS

1 tablespoon olive oil

1 onion, chopped

8 oz mushrooms, sliced

1 1/2 cups Arborio rice

1/2 cup white wine

4 cups vegetable broth

1/2 cup grated Parmesan cheese

Salt and pepper to taste

Fresh parsley for garnish

NUTRITIONAL VALUE

400 calories,

10g protein,

10g fat,

60g carbohydrates,

3g fiber

DIRECTIONS

1. 1. In a large skillet, heat the olive oil over medium heat.
2. 2. Add the onion and cook until softened, about 5 minutes.
3. 3. Add the mushrooms and cook until they release their liquid, about 5 minutes.
4. 4. Add the Arborio rice and cook for another minute, stirring constantly.
5. 5. Add the white wine and cook until it is absorbed.
6. 6. Gradually add the vegetable broth, 1/2 cup at a time, stirring constantly and allowing each addition to be absorbed before adding more.
7. 7. Continue cooking and stirring until the rice is creamy and tender, about 25-30 minutes.
8. 8. Stir in the Parmesan cheese, salt, and pepper.
9. 9. Serve hot, garnished with fresh parsley.

NOTES

This creamy risotto is made with Arborio rice, mushrooms, onions, and Parmesan cheese, perfect for a comforting and satisfying meal.

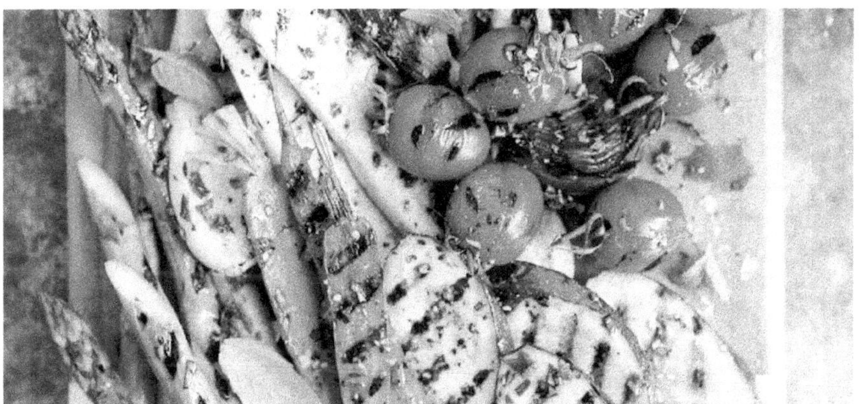

Grilled Vegetable Platter

DIRECTIONS

1.1. Preheat grill to medium-high heat.

2.2. In a large bowl, toss the sliced vegetables with olive oil, salt, and pepper.

3.3. Grill the vegetables for 5-7 minutes per side, or until tender and lightly charred.

4.4. Arrange the grilled vegetables on a platter and drizzle with balsamic glaze.

5.5. Serve hot or at room temperature.

🍴 4 servings 🕐 30 minutes

INGREDIENTS

1 red bell pepper, sliced

1 yellow bell pepper, sliced

1 zucchini, sliced

1 eggplant, sliced

1 bunch asparagus, trimmed

2 tablespoons olive oil

Salt and pepper to taste

Balsamic glaze for serving

NUTRITIONAL VALUE

200 calories,

5g protein,

10g fat,

25g carbohydrates,

8g fiber

NOTES

This vibrant platter is made with a variety of grilled vegetables, such as bell peppers, zucchini, eggplant, and asparagus, served with a tangy balsamic glaze for a flavorful and nutritious meal.

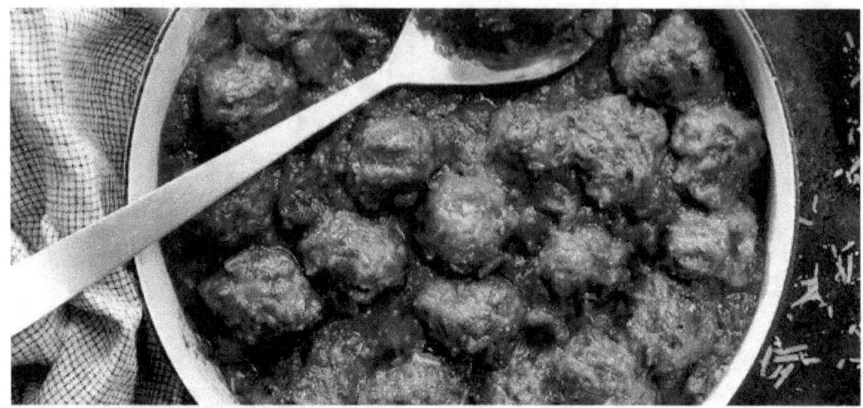

Turkey Meatballs with Marinara Sauce

 4 servings  45 minutes

INGREDIENTS

1 lb ground turkey

1/2 cup breadcrumbs

1/4 cup grated Parmesan cheese

1 teaspoon Italian seasoning

1 egg

Salt and pepper to taste

2 tablespoons olive oil

2 cups marinara sauce

Fresh basil for garnish

NUTRITIONAL VALUE

300 calories,

25g protein,

15g fat,

20g carbohydrates,

3g fiber

DIRECTIONS

1. 1. In a bowl, combine the ground turkey, breadcrumbs, Parmesan cheese, Italian seasoning, egg, salt, and pepper. Mix until well combined.
2. 2. Form the mixture into meatballs.
3. 3. In a large skillet, heat the olive oil over medium heat. Add the meatballs and cook until browned on all sides and cooked through, about 10 minutes.
4. 4. Add the marinara sauce to the skillet and stir to coat the meatballs.
5. 5. Simmer for another 5 minutes.
6. 6. Serve hot, garnished with fresh basil.

NOTES

These turkey meatballs are made with ground turkey, breadcrumbs, Parmesan cheese, and Italian seasoning, served with a homemade marinara sauce for a delicious and satisfying meal.

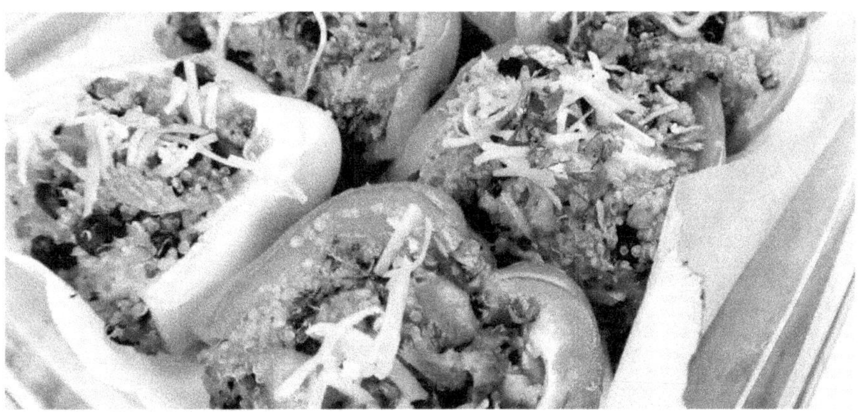

Stuffed Bell Peppers

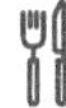 4 servings   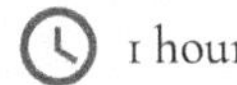 1 hour

INGREDIENTS

4 large bell peppers, halved
and seeded

1 lb ground beef

1 onion, chopped

2 garlic cloves, minced

1 can (14 oz) diced tomatoes

1 cup cooked rice

1 teaspoon dried oregano

1 teaspoon dried basil

Salt and pepper to taste

Shredded cheddar cheese for
topping

NUTRITIONAL VALUE

350 calories,

25g protein,

15g fat,

30g carbohydrates,

5g fiber

DIRECTIONS

1. 1. Preheat oven to 375°F (190°C).
2. 2. Place the bell pepper halves in a baking dish.
3. 3. In a large skillet, cook the ground beef over medium heat until browned. Drain any excess fat.
4. 4. Add the onion and garlic to the skillet. Cook until softened, about 5 minutes.
5. 5. Stir in the diced tomatoes, rice, oregano, basil, salt, and pepper. Cook for another 5 minutes.
6. 6. Spoon the beef mixture into the bell pepper halves.
7. 7. Cover the baking dish with aluminum foil and bake for 30 minutes.
8. 8. Remove the foil, sprinkle the stuffed peppers with shredded cheddar cheese, and bake for another 10 minutes, or until cheese is melted and bubbly.
9. 9. Serve hot.

> **NOTES**
> These stuffed bell peppers are filled with a mixture of ground beef, rice, tomatoes, and spices, then baked to perfection for a satisfying and delicious meal.

Indulgent Desserts

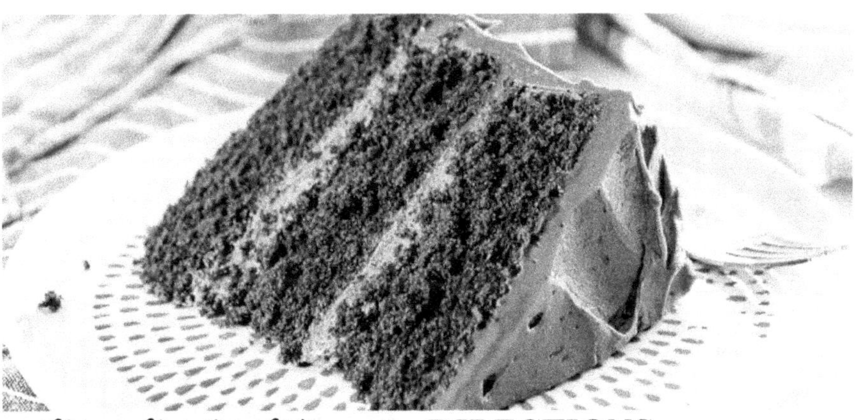

Classic Chocolate Cake

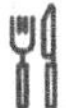 8 servings   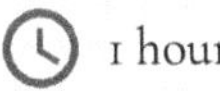 1 hour

INGREDIENTS

1 3/4 cups all-purpose flour

1 1/2 teaspoons baking powder

1 1/2 teaspoons baking soda

1/2 teaspoon salt

3/4 cup unsweetened cocoa
powder

2 cups sugar

1 cup milk

1/2 cup vegetable oil

2 eggs

2 teaspoons vanilla extract

1 cup boiling water

NUTRITIONAL VALUE

400 calories,

5g protein,

15g fat,

65g carbohydrates,

5g fiber

DIRECTIONS

1. 1. Preheat oven to 350°F (175°C). Grease and flour two 9-inch round cake pans.
2. 2. In a large bowl, sift together the flour, baking powder, baking soda, salt, cocoa powder, and sugar.
3. 3. Add the milk, vegetable oil, eggs, and vanilla extract to the dry ingredients. Mix until well combined.
4. 4. Stir in the boiling water. The batter will be thin.
5. 5. Pour the batter evenly into the prepared cake pans.
6. 6. Bake for 30 to 35 minutes, or until a toothpick inserted into the center comes out clean.
7. 7. Cool in the pans for 10 minutes, then remove from pans and cool completely on a wire rack.
8. 8. Frost with your favorite chocolate frosting.

NOTES

This indulgent chocolate cake is moist and rich, perfect for satisfying your chocolate cravings.

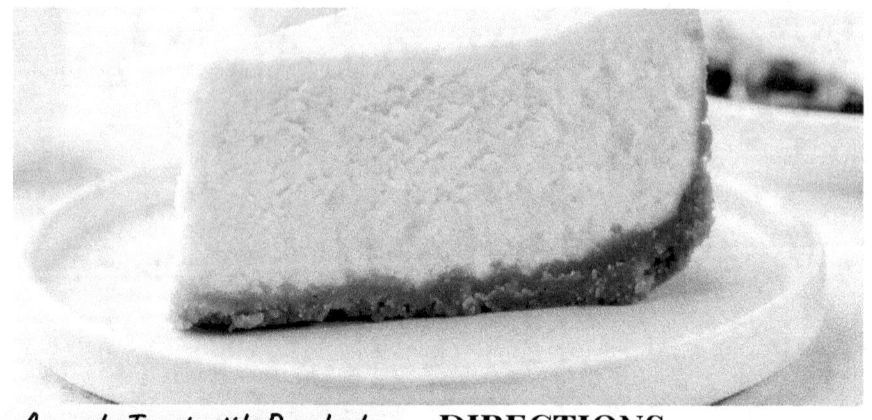

Avocado Toast with Poached Egg

 12 servings 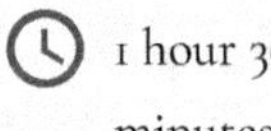 1 hour 30 minutes

INGREDIENTS

1 1/2 cups graham cracker crumbs

1/4 cup sugar

1/2 cup butter, melted

4 (8 oz) packages cream cheese, softened

1 1/4 cups sugar

4 eggs

1 teaspoon vanilla extract

1/2 cup sour cream

1/2 cup heavy cream

NUTRITIONAL VALUE

500 calories,

10g protein,

35g fat,

40g carbohydrates,

1g fiber

DIRECTIONS

1.1. Preheat oven to 325°F (165°C). Grease a 9-inch springform pan.

2.2. In a medium bowl, mix together the graham cracker crumbs, sugar, and melted butter. Press into the bottom of the prepared pan.

3.3. In a large bowl, beat the cream cheese and sugar until smooth. Add the eggs one at a time, mixing well after each addition. Stir in the vanilla extract.

4.4. Pour the cream cheese mixture over the crust.

5.5. Bake for 60 minutes in the preheated oven, or until the center is almost set.

6.6. Turn off the oven and leave the cheesecake in the oven with the door ajar for 1 hour.

7.7. Remove from the oven and cool completely on a wire rack.

8.8. Chill in the refrigerator for at least 4 hours before serving.

NOTES

This classic cheesecake is rich, creamy, and decadent, perfect for special occasions or a delightful treat.

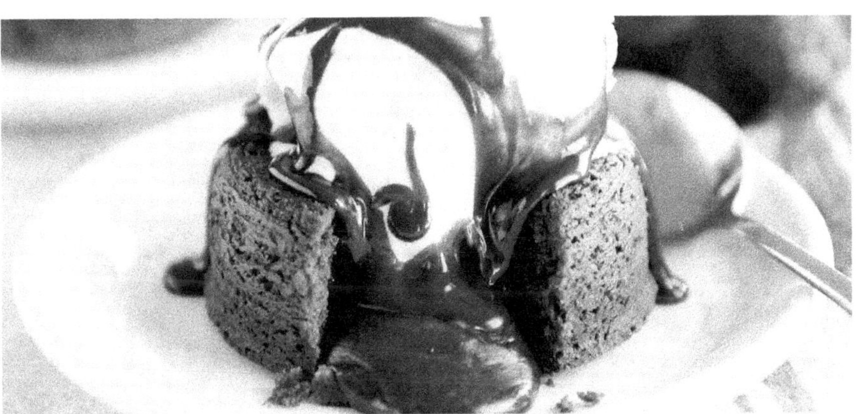

Molten Chocolate Lava Cake

 4 servings   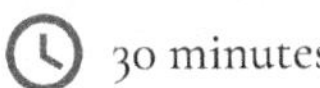 30 minutes

INGREDIENTS

4 oz bittersweet chocolate

1/2 cup unsalted butter

1/4 cup sugar

2 eggs

2 egg yolks

1/2 teaspoon vanilla extract

1/4 cup all-purpose flour

Pinch of salt

Powdered sugar for dusting

NUTRITIONAL VALUE

400 calories,

6g protein,

30g fat,

30g carbohydrates,

2g fiber

DIRECTIONS

1.1. Preheat oven to 450°F (230°C). Grease and flour four 4-ounce ramekins.

2.2. In a medium microwave-safe bowl, melt the chocolate and butter together in the microwave in 30-second intervals, stirring until smooth.

3.3. Whisk in the sugar, eggs, egg yolks, and vanilla extract until well combined.

4.4. Stir in the flour and salt until just combined.

5.5. Divide the batter evenly among the prepared ramekins.

6.6. Bake for 10-12 minutes, or until the edges are set but the center is still soft.

7.7. Remove from the oven and let cool for 1 minute.

8.8. Run a knife around the edges of the cakes to loosen them, then invert onto serving plates.

9.9. Dust with powdered sugar and serve immediately.

NOTES

This indulgent chocolate cake has a gooey, molten center that oozes out when you cut into it, perfect for a luxurious dessert experience.

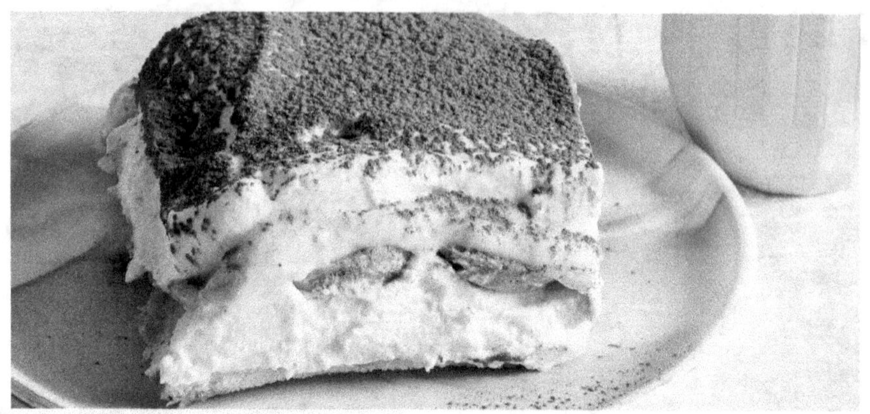

Tiramisu

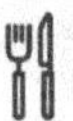 8 servings 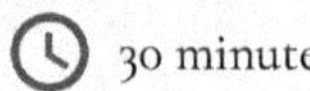 30 minutes

INGREDIENTS

1 cup strong brewed coffee, cooled

3 tablespoons coffee liqueur (optional)

3 eggs, separated

3/4 cup sugar, divided

8 oz mascarpone cheese

1 cup heavy cream

1 teaspoon vanilla extract

24 ladyfinger cookies

Unsweetened cocoa powder for dusting

NUTRITIONAL VALUE

400 calories,

6g protein,

25g fat,

35g carbohydrates,

1g fiber

DIRECTIONS

1. 1. In a shallow dish, combine the coffee and coffee liqueur.
2. 2. In a large bowl, beat the egg yolks and 1/2 cup sugar until thick and pale.
3. 3. Add the mascarpone cheese and beat until smooth.
4. 4. In another bowl, beat the heavy cream, vanilla extract, and remaining 1/4 cup sugar until stiff peaks form.
5. 5. In a separate bowl, beat the egg whites until stiff peaks form.
6. 6. Gently fold the whipped cream into the mascarpone mixture, then fold in the egg whites.
7. 7. Dip each ladyfinger into the coffee mixture briefly, then arrange a layer of ladyfingers in the bottom of a 9x13-inch dish.
8. 8. Spread half of the mascarpone mixture over the ladyfingers.
9. 9. Repeat with another layer of coffee-dipped ladyfingers and the remaining mascarpone mixture.
10. 10. Cover and refrigerate for at least 4 hours, or overnight.
11. 11. Dust with cocoa powder before serving.

NOTES

This classic Italian dessert is made with layers of coffee-soaked ladyfingers and creamy mascarpone cheese, dusted with cocoa powder for a decadent treat.

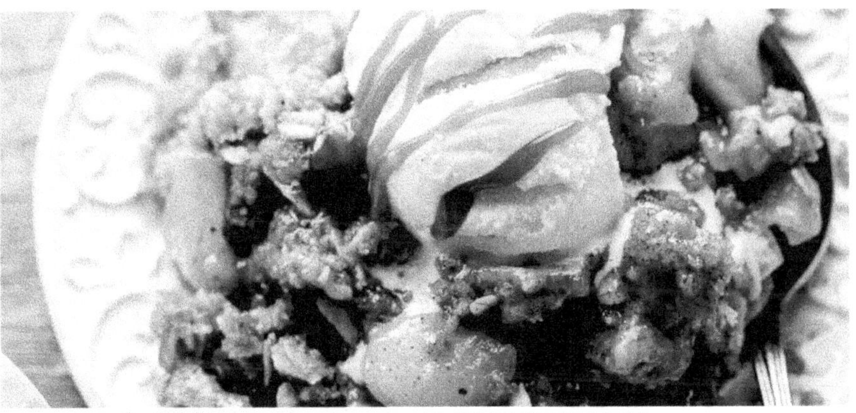

Apple Crisp

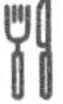 6 servings 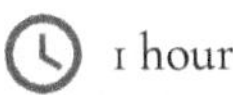 1 hour

INGREDIENTS

4 cups apples, peeled, cored, and sliced

1/2 cup sugar

1 teaspoon cinnamon

1/2 teaspoon nutmeg

1/2 cup all-purpose flour

1/2 cup rolled oats

1/2 cup brown sugar

1/4 cup butter, melted

Vanilla ice cream for serving

NUTRITIONAL VALUE

300 calories,

2g protein,

10g fat,

55g carbohydrates,

4g fiber

DIRECTIONS

1. 1. Preheat oven to 350°F (175°C). Grease a 9-inch baking dish.
2. 2. In a large bowl, combine the apples, sugar, cinnamon, and nutmeg. Spread evenly in the prepared baking dish.
3. 3. In a separate bowl, combine the flour, oats, and brown sugar. Stir in the melted butter until crumbly.
4. 4. Sprinkle the oat mixture over the apples.
5. 5. Bake for 30-35 minutes, or until the apples are tender and the topping is golden brown.
6. 6. Serve warm with vanilla ice cream.

NOTES

This apple crisp is made with tender apples, warm spices, and a crispy oat topping, perfect for a cozy and delicious dessert

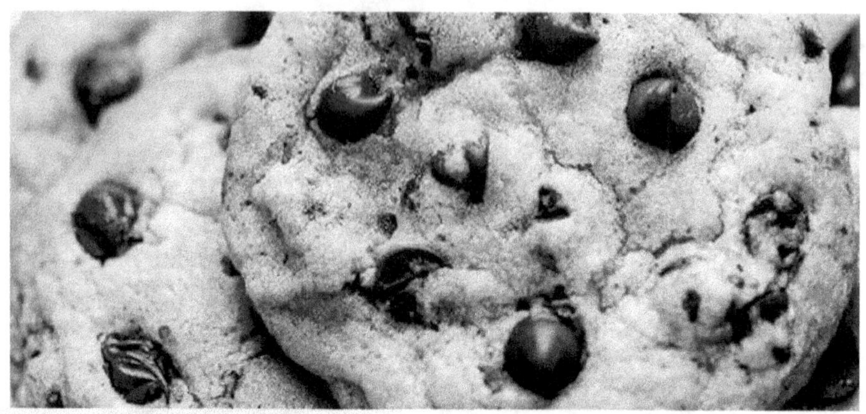

Chocolate Chip Cookies

 24 cookies 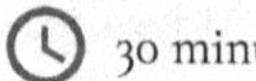 30 minutes

INGREDIENTS

1/2 cup unsalted butter, softened

1/2 cup granulated sugar

1/2 cup brown sugar

1 egg

1 teaspoon vanilla extract

1 1/4 cups all-purpose flour

1/2 teaspoon baking soda

1/2 teaspoon salt

1 cup chocolate chips

NUTRITIONAL VALUE

150 calories,

2g protein,

7g fat,

20g carbohydrates,

1g fiber

DIRECTIONS

1.1. Preheat oven to 350°F (175°C). Line a baking sheet with parchment paper.

2.2. In a large bowl, cream together the butter, granulated sugar, and brown sugar until smooth.

3.3. Beat in the egg and vanilla extract until well blended.

4.4. In a separate bowl, combine the flour, baking soda, and salt. Gradually add to the butter mixture and mix until just blended.

5.5. Stir in the chocolate chips.

6.6. Drop by rounded spoonfuls onto the prepared baking sheet.

7.7. Bake for 8 to 10 minutes, or until light golden brown.

8.8. Cool on the baking sheet for a few minutes before transferring to a wire rack to cool completely.

NOTES

These chocolate chip cookies are soft, chewy, and loaded with chocolate chips, perfect for satisfying your sweet tooth.

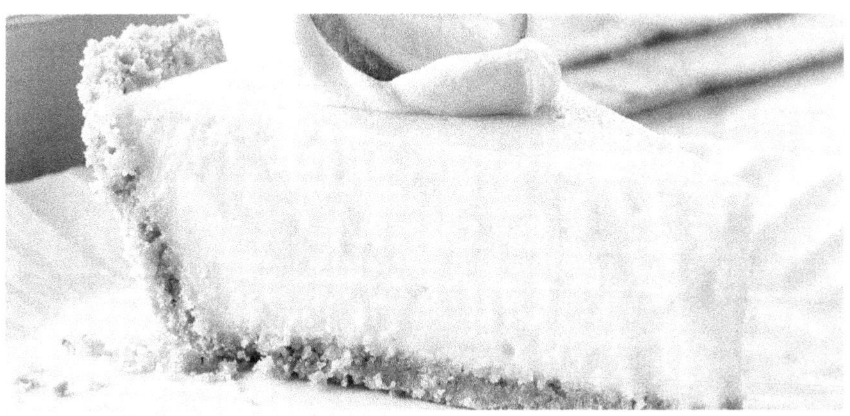

Key Lime Pie

 8 servings 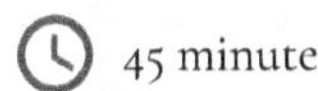 45 minutes

INGREDIENTS

1 1/2 cups graham cracker
crumbs

1/3 cup sugar

6 tablespoons butter, melted

3 egg yolks

1 can (14 oz) sweetened
condensed milk

1/2 cup key lime juice

1 tablespoon key lime zest

Whipped cream for serving

NUTRITIONAL VALUE

350 calories,

7g protein,

15g fat,

45g carbohydrates,

1g fiber

DIRECTIONS

1.1. Preheat oven to 350°F (175°C).

2.2. In a medium bowl, mix together
the graham cracker crumbs, sugar,
and melted butter.

3.3. Press the mixture into the bottom
and up the sides of a 9-inch pie dish.

4.4. Bake the crust for 10 minutes, then
let it cool completely.

5.5. In a large bowl, whisk together the
egg yolks, sweetened condensed
milk, key lime juice, and key lime
zest.

6.6. Pour the mixture into the cooled
crust.

7.7. Bake for 15 minutes, or until the
filling is set.

8.8. Let the pie cool to room
temperature, then refrigerate for at
least 2 hours before serving.

9.9. Serve chilled, topped with whipped
cream.

NOTES

This classic pie is made with fresh key
lime juice, sweetened condensed milk,
and a graham cracker crust, perfect for
a light and tangy treat.

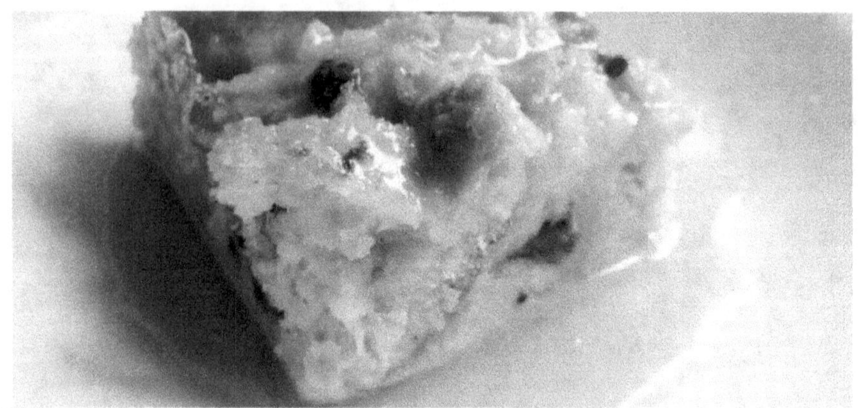

Bread Pudding with Bourbon Sauce

 8 servings    1 hour 30 minutes

INGREDIENTS

1 loaf stale French bread, cut into 1-inch cubes

4 cups milk

1 cup sugar

4 eggs

1 teaspoon vanilla extract

1 teaspoon cinnamon

1/2 teaspoon nutmeg

1/2 cup raisins (optional)

1/2 cup chopped pecans (optional)

1/4 cup butter

1/2 cup sugar

1/4 cup bourbon

NUTRITIONAL VALUE

400 calories,

8g protein,

15g fat,

60g carbohydrates,

2g fiber

DIRECTIONS

1. 1. Preheat oven to 350°F (175°C). Grease a 9x13-inch baking dish.
2. 2. In a large bowl, combine the bread cubes and milk. Let soak for 10 minutes.
3. 3. In another
4. 4. bowl, beat together the sugar, eggs, vanilla extract, cinnamon, and nutmeg.
5. 5. Stir the egg mixture into the bread mixture until well combined.
6. 6. Fold in the raisins and chopped pecans, if using.
7. 7. Pour the mixture into the prepared baking dish.
8. 8. Bake for 45-50 minutes, or until set and golden brown.
9. 9. In a small saucepan, melt the butter over medium heat. Stir in the sugar and bourbon.
10. 10. Bring to a boil, then reduce heat and simmer for 5 minutes, stirring occasionally.
11. 11. Serve the bread pudding warm, drizzled with the bourbon sauce.

NOTES

This bread pudding is made with stale bread, eggs, milk, sugar, and spices, topped with a warm bourbon sauce for a comforting and indulgent treat.

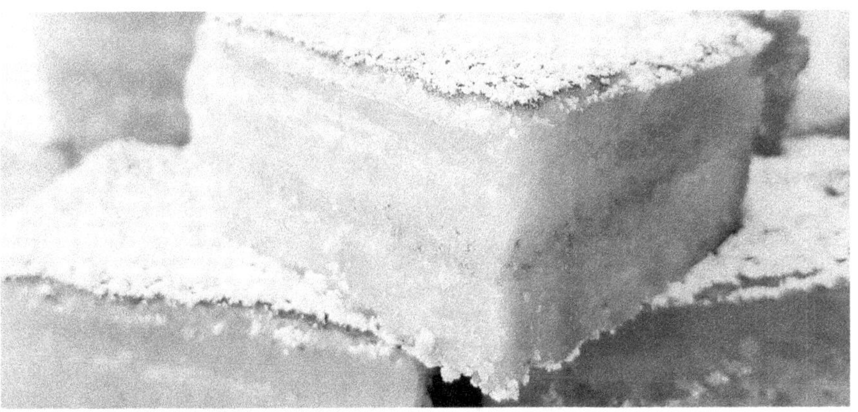

Lemon Bars

 12 bars 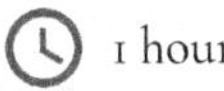 1 hour

INGREDIENTS

1 cup all-purpose flour

1/2 cup powdered sugar

1/2 cup butter, softened

2 eggs

1 cup sugar

2 tablespoons all-purpose flour

1/2 teaspoon baking powder

2 tablespoons lemon juice

1 teaspoon lemon zest

Powdered sugar for dusting

NUTRITIONAL VALUE

200 calories,

2g protein,

10g fat,

30g carbohydrates,

1g fiber

DIRECTIONS

1.1. Preheat oven to 350°F (175°C). Grease a 9x9-inch baking pan.

2.2. In a medium bowl, mix together 1 cup flour and 1/2 cup powdered sugar. Cut in the butter until mixture is crumbly. Press into the prepared pan.

3.3. Bake for 20 minutes, or until firm and golden.

4.4. In another bowl, whisk together the eggs, sugar, 2 tablespoons flour, baking powder, lemon juice, and lemon zest until well combined.

5.5. Pour the lemon mixture over the hot crust.

6.6. Bake for an additional 20-25 minutes, or until the filling is set.

7.7. Cool completely in the pan on a wire rack.

8.8. Dust with powdered sugar before cutting into bars.

NOTES

These lemon bars are made with a buttery shortbread crust and a tangy lemon filling, perfect for a refreshing and citrusy treat.

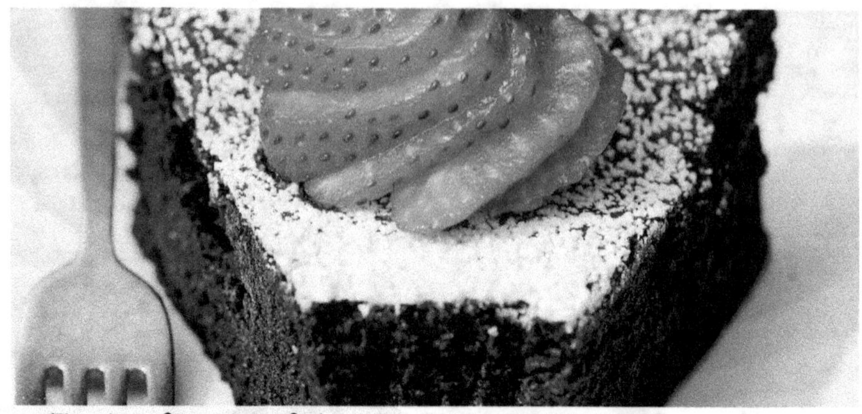

Flourless Chocolate Cake

 8 servings  1 hour

INGREDIENTS

1/2 cup unsalted butter

1 cup semisweet chocolate chips

3/4 cup sugar

1/4 teaspoon salt

1 teaspoon vanilla extract

3 large eggs

1/2 cup unsweetened cocoa powder

Powdered sugar for dusting

NUTRITIONAL VALUE

400 calories,

6g protein,

25g fat,

40g carbohydrates,

3g fiber

DIRECTIONS

1. 1. Preheat oven to 375°F (190°C). Grease an 8-inch round cake pan and line with parchment paper.
2. 2. In a small saucepan, melt the butter and chocolate chips together over low heat, stirring until smooth. Remove from heat and let cool slightly.
3. 3. In a large bowl, whisk together the sugar, salt, vanilla extract, and eggs until well combined.
4. 4. Whisk in the melted chocolate mixture until smooth.
5. 5. Sift the cocoa powder over the batter and fold in until no streaks remain.
6. 6. Pour the batter into the prepared pan and smooth the top.
7. 7. Bake for 20-25 minutes, or until a toothpick inserted into the center comes out with moist crumbs.
8. 8. Let the cake cool in the pan for 10 minutes, then invert onto a wire rack to cool completely.
9. 9. Dust with powdered sugar before serving.

NOTES

This flourless chocolate cake is dense, fudgy, and intensely chocolatey, perfect for a luxurious dessert experience.

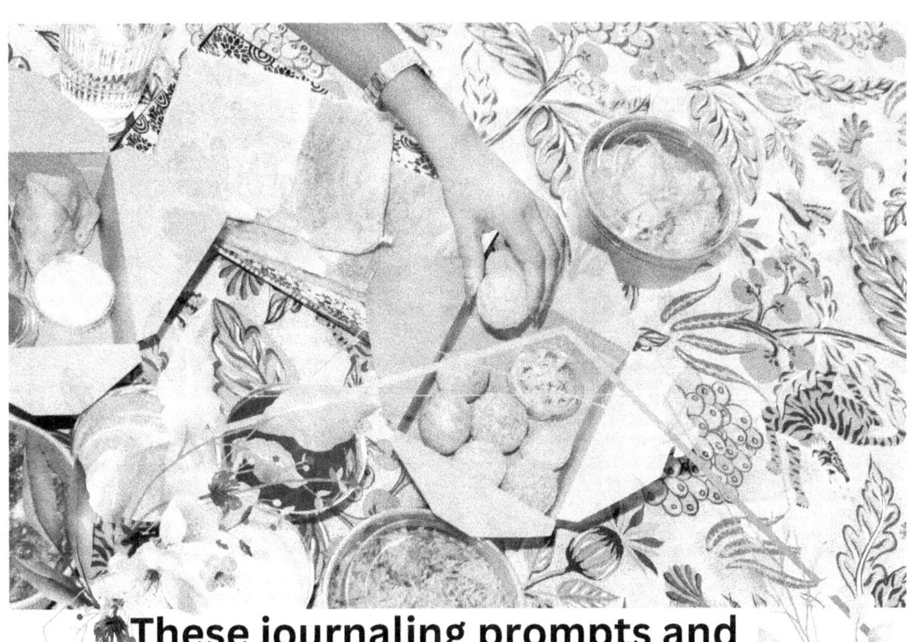

These journaling prompts and activities are designed to encourage reflection, mindfulness, and self-awareness when it comes to food and eating habits.

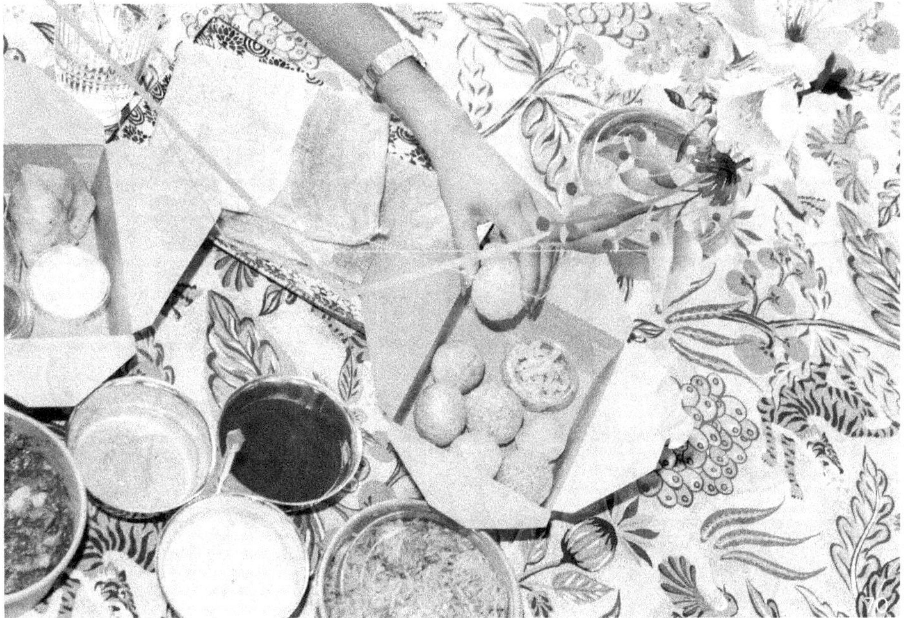

Write about a food that brings you comfort and why. How does it make you feel when you eat it?

Describe a meal that you enjoyed recently. What made it special? How did you feel before, during, and after eating?

Write about a food memory from your childhood. How does this memory influence your relationship with food today?

Describe a time when you ate something purely for pleasure. What did you eat? How did it taste? How did you feel afterwards?

List three ways you can practice self-care that don't involve food. How do these activities make you feel?

Write a letter to your body, thanking it for all that it does for you. Express gratitude for its strength, resilience, and beauty.

Think about a food rule that you follow. Is it serving you well? How does it impact your relationship with food?

Describe a time when you felt guilty about eating something. What triggered this feeling? How did you respond?

List three ways you can incorporate more mindful eating into your daily life. How do you think this will benefit you?

Reflect on a time when you felt judged for your food choices. How did it make you feel? How did you respond?

List three foods that you've labeled as "good" and three foods that you've labeled as "bad." Challenge these labels and explore the idea of food neutrality.

Reflect on a time when you felt out of control around food. What triggered this feeling? How did you cope?

Describe a meal that you would consider "balanced." What does balance mean to you when it comes to food?

List three things you can do to cultivate a positive relationship with food and your body. How can you incorporate these practices into your daily life?

Conclusion

The Intuitive Eating Cookbook" offers a holistic approach to food and eating, focusing on listening to your body's hunger and fullness cues, and enjoying food without guilt or restriction. By rejecting the diet mentality and embracing intuitive eating principles, you can develop a healthy and balanced relationship with food.

Through the recipes in this cookbook, you can learn to honor your hunger, make peace with food, challenge the food police, and discover the satisfaction factor in eating. You'll find a variety of delicious and nutritious recipes that cater to different tastes and preferences, ensuring that eating intuitively is not only nourishing but also enjoyable.

By incorporating the principles of intuitive eating into your life and using this cookbook as a guide, you can learn to cope with your feelings without using food, respect your body, and honor your health through gentle nutrition. This book is not just about what you eat, but how you eat, promoting a mindful and joyful approach to food that can enhance your overall well-being.

"The Intuitive Eating Cookbook" is not just a collection of recipes but a journey towards a healthier relationship with food and yourself. It encourages you to trust your body's wisdom and embrace a positive and sustainable approach to eating that can benefit you for years to come.

www.ingramcontent.com/pod-product-compliance
Lightning Source LLC
Chambersburg PA
CBHW050833260726
48660CB00006B/2212